C000296748

Author: Debabrata Mukherjee, MD, Tyler Gill Professor of Interventional Cardiology
Gill Heart Institute, Division of Cardiovascular Medicine, University of Kentucky
Editor: Carla Maute, M.D.
Cover Illustration: Lucy Mikyna
Production: Sylvia Engel
Publisher: Börm Bruckmeier Publishing LLC, www.media4u.com

© 2006, by **Börm Bruckmeier Publishing LLC**
68 17th Street, Hermosa Beach, CA 90254
www.media4u.com
First Edition

IMPORTANT NOTICE – PLEASE READ!
This book is based on information from sources believed to be reliable, and every effort has been
made to make the book as complete and accurate as possible and to describe generally accepted
practices based on information available as of the printing date, but its accuracy and completeness
cannot be guaranteed. Despite the best efforts of authors, editors and publisher, the book may
contain errors, and the reader should use the book only as a general guide and not as the ultimate
source of information about the subject matter.
This book is not intended to reprint all of the information available to the author or
publisher on the subject, but rather to simplify, complement and supplement other available
sources. The reader is encouraged to read all available material and to consult the package
insert and other references to learn as much as possible about the subject.
This book is sold without warranties of any kind, expressed or implied, and the publisher and
author disclaim any liability, loss or damage caused by the content of this book.
IF YOU DO NOT WISH TO BE BOUND BY THE FOREGOING CAUTIONS AND CONDITIONS , YOU
MAY RETURN THIS BOOK TO THE PUBLISHER FOR A FULL REFUND.

Printed in China
ISBN 1-59103-229-6

Preface

A 12-lead ECG is a simple, inexpensive, non-invasive test that can provide a wealth of clinical information about the patient and is typically one of the first tests carried out on a medical patient in the hospital setting. It is imperative for residents, fellows, emergency room physicians, and hospitalists to be able to interpret major abnormalities in the ECG quickly and accurately. It is therefore essential that clinicians are familiar with common ECG morphologies or typical ECG patterns seen in a particular pathology or clinical condition.

The **ECG Cases pocket** provides examples of common clinical problems encountered in the wards, emergency room, or outpatient setting to enable the clinician to quickly and accurately recognize ECG morphologies that will guide further patient management. Subtle or unusual ECG findings are not presented, and are not the focus of this text.

Each ECG is preceded by a brief clinical history and pertinent physical examination findings, so that the tracings may be interpreted in the appropriate clinical context.

The convenient size of this book will enable medical students, interns, residents, and other trainees to carry it in their pockets, for use as a quick reference against which to compare ECG patterns they may encounter.

Finally, the major ECG diagnoses are identified by the **American Board of Internal Medicine (ABIM) code**, which should be very helpful for trainees preparing for the Internal Medicine, Family Medicine, and Cardiovascular Medicine Boards, or other certifying examinations.

I anticipate that this book will help clinicians to identify common ECG abnormalities encountered in practice, and will ultimately improve patient care.

D. Mukherjee   February, 2006

All ECGs in this booklet are
recorded at a speed of 25 mm/sec.

Scaling factor of the ECGs is 75%.

Börm Bruckmeier Publishing LLC on the Internet:
www.media4u.com

Contents

6 Contents

Drug pocket plus

A must for students, residents and all other healthcare professionals

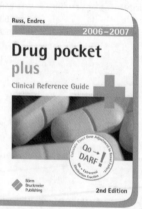

Russ, Endres

2006–2007

Drug pocket
plus

Clinical Reference Guide

Q0 → DARF !

Börm
Bruckmeier
Publishing

2nd Edition

ISBN 1-59103-226-1   US $ 24.95

- This pocket book conveniently combines the contents of the best selling **Drug pocket** and the **Drug Therapy pocket** in one volume

- Contains more than 1,200 **drugs** and approximately **2,300 brand names**

- Contains **prescription requirements** and prescribing information for each individual drug

- Provides treatment regimens for more than 230 medical conditions

- Uses a clever system of cross-referencing between the drug therapy sections and the drug information sections

- Now includes the equation for precise calculation of dose adjustments in renal failure

Contents: types of condition, as coded by the ABIM

45. Left anterior fascicular block	Case 27, Case 38, Case 43
	Case 46, Case 52
46. Left posterior fascicular block	no case
47. Left bundle branch block, complete	Case 10
48. Left bundle branch block, incomplete	no case
49. Intraventricular conduction disturbance, non-specific type	Case 3
	Case 32, Case 49
	Case 52, Case 54
50. Functional (rate-relat.) aberrant intraventric. conduction	Case 51

Q Wave Myocardial Infarction

51. Anterolateral myocardial infarction, age recent or probably acute	Case 31
52. Anterolateral myocardial infarction, age indeterminate or probably old	no case
53. Anterior or anteroseptal myocardial infarction, age recent or probably acute	no case
54. Anterior or anteroseptal myocardial infarction, age indeterminate or probably old	Case 49
55. Lateral myocardial infarction, age recent or probably acute	Case 32
56. Lateral myocardial infarction, age indeterminate or probably old	no case
57. Inferior myocardial infarction, age recent or probably acute	Case 8, Case 32, Case 56
58. Inferior myocardial infarction, age indeterminate or probably old	Case 54
59. Posterior myocardial infarction, age recent or probably acute	Case 33
60. Posterior myocardial infarction, age indeterminate or probably old	Case 54

ST, T, U Wave Abnormalities

61. Normal variant, early repolarization	Case 5
62. Normal variant, juvenile T waves	no case
63. Non-specific ST segment and/or T wave abnormalities	Case 1
	Case 3, Case 4, Case 6
	Case 7, Case 27
64. ST segment and/or T wave abnormalities suggesting myocardial ischemia	Case 13, Case 30, Case 37

Case 1

1.1   Clinical Scenario

A 53-year-old female presents to your office with shortness of breath which began four hours earlier. She returned from a long road trip two days ago and was doing well prior to the development of her current symptoms. She denies having any chest pain. Her past medical history is significant for diet-controlled type II diabetes mellitus and hypertension. Her medications include thiazide diuretics for hypertension and hormone replacement therapy. On physical examination, she appears diaphoretic and in moderate respiratory distress. She is afebrile, has a heart rate of 146 beats/minute, a respiratory rate of 26/minute and a blood pressure of 164/96 mmHg. Her cardiac examination reveals a mildly elevated jugular venous pressure and cardiac examination reveals an S4 gallop and a soft Grade I/VI systolic murmur. Her lungs are clear to auscultation.

1.2   Questions

1. What is the most likely diagnosis?

2. What should be the next diagnostic test?

3. What does the ECG show?

4. What is the optimal treatment for this patient?

1.3 ECG Sample

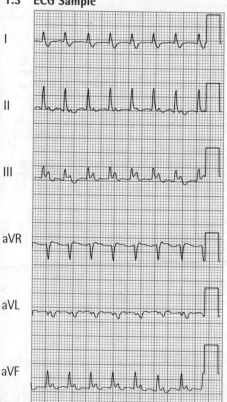

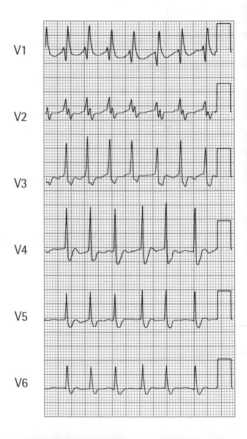

1.4   Answers

1. The most likely diagnosis is acute pulmonary embolism (PE) given her recent road trip and use of hormone replacement therapy. Other possibilities include acute pneumothorax, pneumonia, angina pectoris equivalent and pulmonary edema.

2. The initial diagnostic test should be an ECG, but ECG findings are often non-specific in acute PE. The ECG is often more helpful in excluding other diagnoses. The most common ECG abnormalities in PE are sinus tachycardia and non-specific ST-T wave abnormalities. Other ECG findings of right heart strain, such as peaked P waves in lead II (P pulmonale), right-axis deviation, right bundle branch block, an S1-Q3-T3 pattern, or atrial fibrillation may be seen, but < 20% of patients with proven PE have any of these classic ECG abnormalities.

3. The 12-lead ECG shows irregularly irregular rhythm due to **atrial fibrillation** [ABIM code # 19], right bundle branch block [ABIM code # 43] and non-specific ST segment and/or T wave changes [ABIM code # 63]. All of these findings are consistent with a diagnosis of acute PE.

4. Early heparin anticoagulation is imperative, and heparin should be started as soon as the diagnosis of PE is considered. Anticoagulation should not wait for the results of diagnostic tests because if anti-coagulation is delayed, venous thrombosis and PE may progress rapidly. Fibrinolysis is indicated for patients with PE who have evidence of right heart strain, because the mortality rate can be significantly reduced by early fibrinolysis in this patient population.

Case 2

2.1 Clinical Scenario

A 23-year-old male is referred to you for further evaluation after an abnormal ECG during a routine physical examination. He denies having any cardiac symptoms and does not have any significant medical history. On examination, he appears comfortable without any acute distress. He is afebrile, has a heart rate of 88 beats/minute, respiratory rate of 12/minute and a blood pressure of 128/72 mmHg. His cardiac examination reveals normal heart sounds without any rub, gallop, or murmur, and the lungs are clear to auscultation.

2.2 Questions

1. What does the ECG show?

2. What should you do next?

2.3 ECG Sample

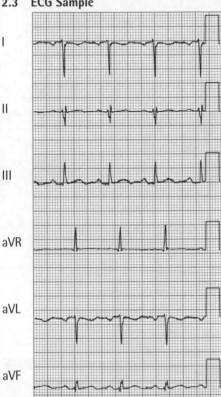

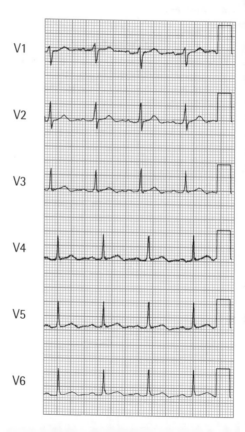

2.4   Answers

1. The 12-lead ECG shows normal sinus rhythm [ABIM code # 7] with **limb lead reversal** [ABIM code # 3], which may mimic a lateral myocardial infarction.

2. A repeat ECG with correct electrode placement showed normal sinus rhythm with a normal ECG. The patient was reassured without further diagnostic tests.

Case 3

3.1 Clinical Scenario

A 64-year-old female presents to your office with palpitations and lightheadedness which began six hours earlier. She also complains of some vague chest discomfort. Her past medical history is significant for hyperlipidemia and hypertension. Her medications include atenolol for hypertension and atorvastatin for hyperlipidemia. On physical examination, she appears uncomfortable but is not in acute distress. She is afebrile, has a heart rate of 52 beats/minute, respiratory rate of 14/minute and a blood pressure of 148/88 mmHg. Her cardiac examination reveals a mildly elevated jugular venous pressure, and cardiac examination reveals a Grade II/VI systolic murmur. Her lungs are clear to auscultation.

3.2 Questions

1. What is the most likely diagnosis?

2. What should be the next diagnostic test?

3. What does the ECG show?

4. What is the optimal tratment for this patient?

3.3 ECG Sample

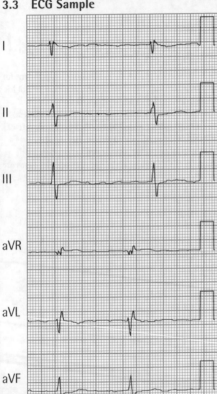

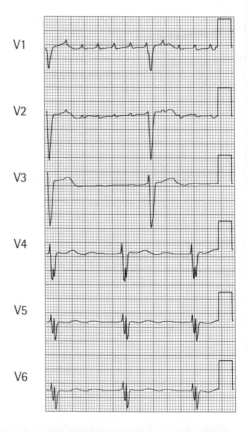

3.4 Answers

1. The most likely diagnosis in someone presenting with palpitations and lightheadedness is a cardiac dysrhythmia.

2. The initial diagnostic test should be a 12-lead ECG. If the ECG on presentation is normal in patients with paroxysmal arrhythmia a Holter monitor or an event recorder may identify the underlying arrhythmia.

3. The 12-lead ECG shows an irregularly irregular rhythm due to **atrial flutter** [ABIM code # 18] with variable atrioventricular (AV) conduction, a nonspecific intraventricular conduction disturbance [ABIM code # 49], and non-specific ST segment and/or T wave changes [ABIM code # 63]. Atrial rate during typical type I atrial flutter is usually 250-350 beats/minute, although class IA and IC antiarrhythmic drugs and amiodarone can reduce the rate to approximately 200 beats/minute. A significantly slower ventricular rate in the absence of drugs suggests abnormal AV conduction.

4. If the patient is unstable with atrial flutter or fibrillation (e.g. hypotension, pulmonary edema, angina), synchronous direct-current (DC) cardioversion is commonly the initial treatment of choice. Cardioversion often requires low energies (<50 J). If the electrical shock results in atrial fibrillation, a second shock at a higher energy level may then be used to restore normal sinus rhythm (NSR). To slow the ventricular response in patients with tachycardia, beta-blockers or calcium channel blockers may be used. Adenosine produces transient AV block and can be used to reveal flutter waves if the diagnosis is in question. In this patient with relative bradycardia most likely due to a combination of being on beta-blockers and intrinsic abnormality in AV conduction, rate control was not an issue. Most patients with atrial flutter can be cured with ablation and this patient underwent flutter ablation as well as placement of a DDDR pacemaker due to underlying sick sinus syndrome. Patients with atrial flutter should be anti-coagulated similarly to patients with atrial fibrillation.

Case 4

4.1 Clinical Scenario

A 44-year-old female librarian presents to your office with a history of palpitations for several weeks. She denies having any angina or other cardiac symptoms, despite regular, moderate regular physical exercise. She has taken her own pulse, which she thought was irregular, and is very concerned about having this condition known as "atrial fibrillation", which she has read may lead to stroke. On physical examination, she appears comfortable and in no acute distress. She is afebrile, has an irregular heart rate of 80-150 beats/minute, respiratory rate of 14/minute and a blood pressure of 163/94 mmHg. Her cardiac examination reveals irregular heart rhythm and no other cardiac abnormality. Her lungs are clear to auscultation.

4.2 Questions

1. What is the most likely diagnosis?

2. What should be the next diagnostic test?

3. What does the ECG show?

4. What is the optimal treatment for this patient?

4.3 ECG Sample

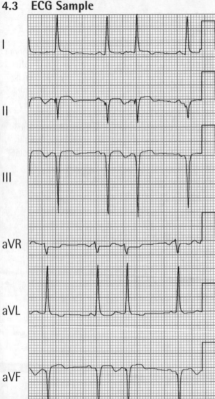

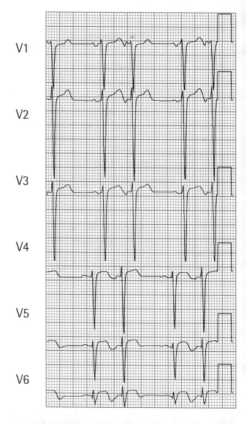

4.4   Answers

1. Conditions that can cause palpitations with an irregular pulse
    include atrial fibrillation, atrial flutter with variable atrioventricular
    conduction, and multiple premature atrial and/or ventricular ectopics.

2. The initial diagnostic test should be a 12-lead ECG. If the ECG on
    presentation is normal in patients with paroxysmal arrhythmia, a Holter
    monitor or an event recorder may identify the underlying arrhythmia.

3. The 12-lead ECG shows normal sinus rhythm [ABIM code # 7],
    atrial premature complexes [ABIM code # 13], left-axis deviation
    [ABIM code # 37], left ventricular hypertrophy [ABIM code # 40] and
    non-specific ST segment and/or T wave abnormalities [ABIM code
    # 63]. The ECG meets the CORNELL voltage criteria for left ventricular
    hypertrophy:

    "S in V3 + R in aVL > 24 mm (men)
    "S in V3 + R in aVL > 20 mm (women)

4. The patient needs to be reassured that she does not have atrial
    fibrillation and that the irregular rhythm is due to multiple extra beats.
    She needs to be treated appropriately for hypertension since an
    enlarged left atrium may be contributing to the multiple ectopics.
    A beta-blocker may treat her hypertension adequately and will also
    decrease the frequency of the premature beats.

Case 5

5.1 Clinical Scenario

A 16-year-old male is referred to you for evaluation of chest pain.
He recently helped his girlfriend move house and lifted several heavy
boxes for her. The discomfort is on both sides of the chest and feels like
a dull ache. He denies having any cardiac symptoms and does not have
any significant medical history. On physical examination, he appears
comfortable without any acute distress. He is afebrile, has a heart rate
of 88 beats/minute, respiratory rate of 12/minute and a blood pressure
of 111/73 mmHg. His cardiac examination reveals normal heart sounds
without any rub, gallop or murmur and the lungs are clear to
auscultation.

5.2 Questions

1. What does the ECG show?

2. What should you do next?

5.3 ECG Sample

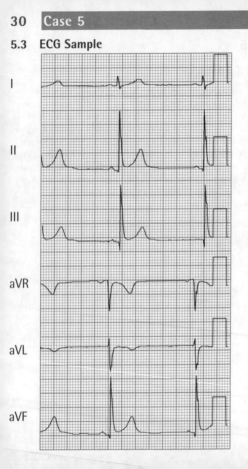

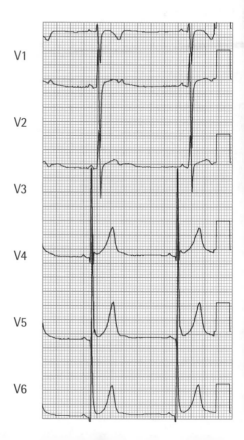

5.4 Answers

1. The 12-lead ECG shows normal sinus rhythm [ABIM code # 7] with **early repolarization** [ABIM code # 61], which may mimic myocardial injury. It may be due to late depolarization and may be a very normal finding, even up to 3-4 mm in amplitude. Normally, early repolarization lessens with increases in heart rate, while ischemic ST segment elevation increases. The ST segment elevation in V4-6 is concave upwards, another characteristic of this normal variant.

2. The patient should be given a copy of his 12-lead ECG to carry around with him so that if he has chest pain in the future he is not misdiagnosed as having an acute myocardial infarction.

Case 6

6.1   Clinical Scenario

You are asked to see a 58-year-old male for an abnormal heart rhythm. He underwent repair of an abdominal aortic aneurysm two days ago. On physical examination, he is afebrile, and has a heart rate of 186 beats/minute and blood pressure of 78/49 mmHg. Lung examination reveals bibasilar rales. You order a 12-lead ECG and a complete metabolic panel.

6.2   Questions

1.   What does the ECG show?

2.   How should he be treated?

6.3 ECG Sample

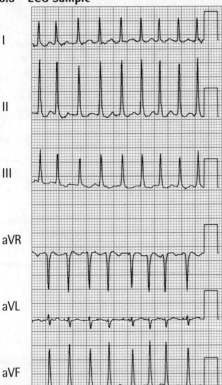

I

II

III

aVR

aVL

aVF

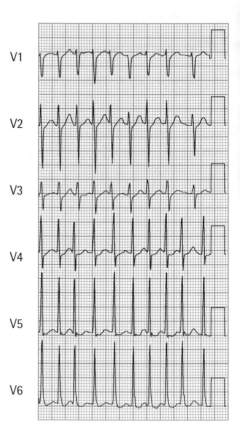

6.4   Answers

1. The 12-lead ECG shows **atrial fibrillation** [ABIM code # 19] with a rapid ventricular rate and non-specific ST segment and/or T wave abnormalities [ABIM code # 63].

2. A patient with new-onset atrial fibrillation who is stable may benefit from simple rate-control measures (e.g. beta-blockers, calcium channel blockers). Unstable patients with hypotension, pulmonary edema, or heart failure should be cardioverted immediately. This patient was successfully cardioverted with 200 J with improvement in his blood pressure and pulmonary edema. Long-term management should include evaluation for cardiac ischemia, left ventricular function, and anticoagulation.

Case 7

7.1 Clinical Scenario

A 57-year-old female presents to your office for routine evaluation. She has not had any prior cardiac symptoms and denies having angina, dyspnea, or orthopnea. She admits to having occasional palpitations. On physical examination, she is afebrile, has a heart rate of 86 beats/minute, respiratory rate of 12/minute and a blood pressure of 133/65 mmHg. Her cardiac examination reveals a soft, Grade I/VI systolic murmur. You request a 12 lead ECG.

7.2 Questions

1. What does the ECG show?

2. What is the optimal treatment for this patient?

7.3 ECG Sample

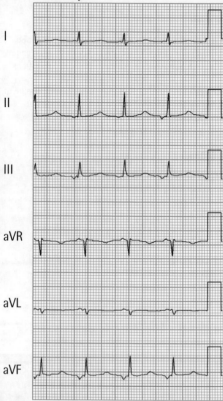

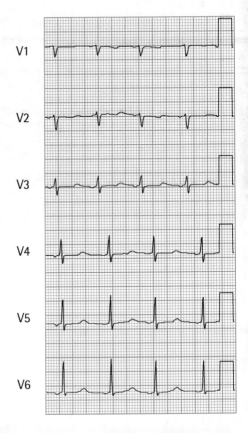

7.4 Answers

1. The 12-lead ECG shows **atrial tachycardia** [ABIM code # 15], with non-specific ST segment and/or T wave changes [ABIM code # 63].

2. Several options are available for the treatment of patients with ectopic atrial tachycardia, including medication to suppress the arrhythmia or control the ventricular response, surgery, or radiofrequency (RF) ablation. Medical therapy is effective in most patients. RF ablation has been very successful in curing atrial tachycardia, with success rates close to 100% and is now the treatment of choice for symptomatic patients. Asymptomatic individuals such as this patient may not need any particular therapy but may potentially benefit from beta-blockers.

Case 8

8.1   Clinical Scenario

A 79-year-old male comes to the emergency room with weakness, fatigue, and chest heaviness. His past medical history is significant for coronary artery disease, with prior stent insertion his right coronary artery. On physical examination, he appears lethargic. He is afebrile, has a heart rate of 52 beats/minute, respiratory rate of 14/minute and a blood pressure of 79/44 mmHg. His cardiac examination reveals a Grade I/VI systolic murmur. You request a 12-lead ECG.

8.2   Questions

1.   What does the ECG show?

2.   What is the optimal treatment for this patient?

8.3 ECG Sample

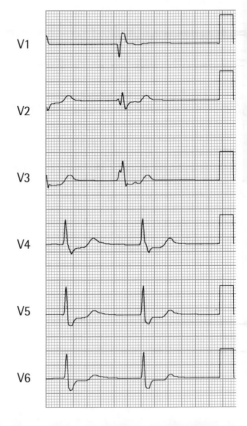

8.4 Answers

1. The 12-lead ECG shows **junctional rhythm** [ABIM code # 22] and underlying acute inferior wall myocardial infarction with ST segment elevation in leads II, III, and aVF [ABIM code # 57].

2. For patients with ST segment elevation on the 12-lead ECG, reperfusion therapy should be initiated as soon as possible, without waiting for cardiac biomarker results. This patient should preferably be sent to the cardiac catheterization laboratory for primary angioplasty; if such facilities are not available and the likely transfer time is more than 60 minutes, fibrinolytics should be administered. If immediately available, primary percutaneous coronary intervention (PCI) should be performed in patients with ST segment elevation myocardial infarction (including true posterior myocardial infarction) or myocardial infarction with new or presumably new left bundle branch block (LBBB) who can undergo percutaneous coronary intervention of the infarct artery within 12 hours of symptom onset, if performed in a timely fashion (balloon inflation within 90 minutes of presentation) by persons skilled in the procedure. This patient has symptomatic junctional bradycardia and needs a temporary transvenous pacemaker.

Case 9

9.1 Clinical Scenario

A 33-year-old female comes to the emergency room with chest pain, which began three days ago. She recently had an upper respiratory tract infection but is otherwise healthy. Her chest discomfort is worse with respiration. On physical examination, she has a heart rate of 119 beats/minute, respiratory rate of 14/minute and a blood pressure of 139/84 mmHg. Her cardiac examination reveals a scratchy sound over the left lower sternal edge. You request a 12-lead ECG.

9.2 Questions

1. What does the ECG show?

2. What is the optimal treatment for this patient?

9.3 ECG Sample

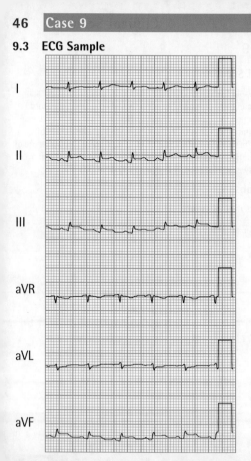

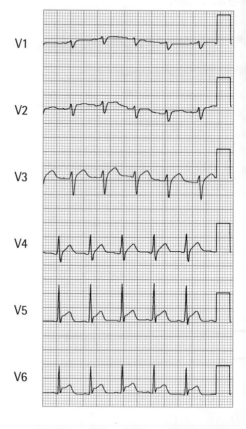

9.4 Answers

1. The 12-lead ECG shows diffuse concave upward ST segment elevation, except aVR and V1 (usually depressed), upright T waves in the leads with ST segment elevation, and PR segment deviation opposite to P wave polarity consistent with acute **pericarditis** [ABIM code # 84], and sinus tachycardia [ABIM code # 10].

2. Treatment for specific causes of pericarditis is directed to the underlying cause. For patients with idiopathic or viral pericarditis, such as our patient, therapy is directed at symptom relief with non-steroidal anti-inflammatory agents.

Case 10

10.1 Clinical Scenario

A 67-year-old male presents to your office for cardiac evaluation. His past medical history is significant for hypertension, coronary artery disease, and chronic obstructive pulmonary disease (COPD). His medications include atenolol, thiazide diuretics, and nitrates. On physical examination, he appears comfortable, and in no acute distress. He is afebrile, has a heart rate of 50 beats/minute, a respiratory rate of 14/minute and a blood pressure of 119/65 mmHg. His cardiac examination reveals split heart sounds without a gallop, rub or murmur. You request a 12-lead ECG and a lipid profile.

10.2 Questions

1. What does the ECG show?

2. What is the optimal treatment for this patient?

10.3 ECG Sample

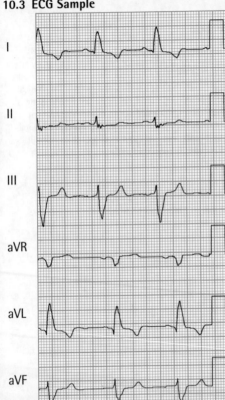

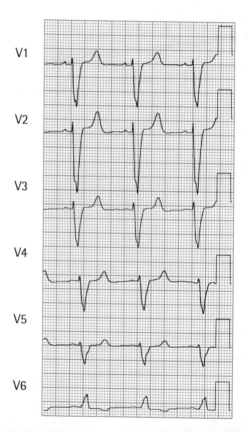

10.4 Answers

1. The 12-lead ECG shows sinus rhythm [ABIM code # 7] and **complete left bundle branch block (LBBB)** [ABIM code # 47]. Complete LBBB has a QRS duration > 0.12 seconds. Terminal S waves in lead V1 indicate late posterior forces, and terminal R waves in leads I, aVL, and V6 indicate late leftward forces. Typically, broad, monophasic R waves are seen in leads I, aVL, and V6 and poor R progression from V1 to V3. ST-T segments in LBBB should be oriented opposite to the direction of the terminal QRS forces (i.e. in leads with terminal R or R' forces, the ST-T segments should be downwards; in leads with terminal S forces the ST-T segments should be upwards). If the ST-T waves are in the same direction or concordant as the terminal QRS forces, they should be labeled primary ST-T wave abnormalities and is suggestive of ischemia.

2. LBBB usually indicates underlying cardiac pathology and is seen in dilated cardiomyopathy, hypertrophic cardiomyopathy, hypertension, aortic valve disease, coronary artery disease, and a variety of other cardiac conditions. In patients who have heart failure from dilated cardiomyopathy and bundle branch block, resynchronization pacing may improve myocardial function. In asymptomatic individuals, no further therapy is indicated, except regular follow-up.

Case 11

11.1 Clinical Scenario

A 37-year-old female presents to the emergency room with generalized weakness, fatigue, and lethargy. She has had a stomach virus for the past four days and has had several bouts of emesis and watery diarrhea. She is afebrile, has a heart rate of 90 beats/minute, respiratory rate of 16/minute and a blood pressure of 89/65 mmHg. Her cardiac examination reveals normal heart sounds without a gallop, rub or murmur. You request a 12-lead ECG and a complete metabolic panel.

11.2 Questions

1. What does the ECG show?

2. What is the optimal treatment for this patient?

11.3 ECG Sample

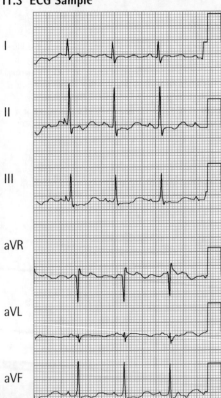

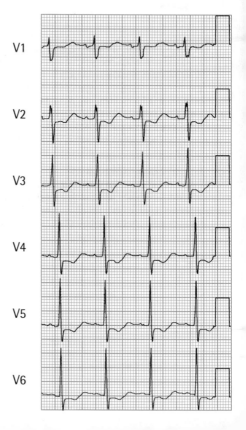

11.4 Answers

1. The 12-lead ECG shows sinus rhythm [ABIM code # 7], T wave flattening with inverted T waves, prominent U waves that appear as QT prolongation, and ST segment depression - all of which are consistent with **hypokalemia** [ABIM code # 75]. The ECG patterns seen in patients with hypokalemia range from mild T wave flattening to the appearance of prominent U waves, occasionally with ST segment depressions or T wave inversions. When the U wave is greater than the T wave, the potassium level is usually lower than 2.5 mEq/L. Hypokalemia may also cause atrial and ventricular arrhythmias. This patient's potassium level was 2.1 mEq/L consistent with severe hypokalemia.

2. Patients in whom severe hypokalemia is suspected should be placed on a cardiac monitor, and an intravenous line placed. Potassium should be administered at 10-20 mEq/h IV via a peripheral or central line. Serum potassium is difficult to replenish if serum magnesium is also low, and the magnesium level should be checked in all patients with hypokalemia.

Case 12

12.1 Clinical Scenario

You are asked to see a 52-year-old male in the hospital for cardiac arrhythmias. He was admitted to the hospital for aortic aneurysm surgery, and his post-operative course has been complicated by renal dysfunction. His past medical history is significant for hypertension, hyperlipidemia, peripheral arterial disease, and type II diabetes mellitus. On physical examination, he appears drowsy and lethargic. He is afebrile, has a heart rate of 35 beats/minute, a respiratory rate of 14/minute, and a blood pressure of 107/66 mmHg. His cardiac examination reveals a Grade II/VI systolic murmur. You request a 12-lead ECG and a complete metabolic panel.

12.2 Questions

1. What does the ECG show?

2. What is the optimal treatment for this patient?

12.3 ECG Sample

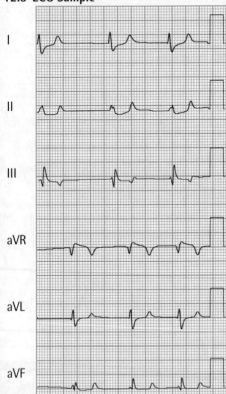

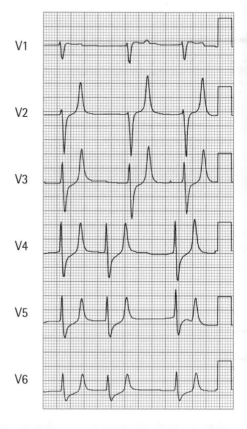

12.4 Answers

1. The 12-lead ECG shows atrial fibrillation [ABIM code # 19], right-axis deviation [ABIM code 38], and peaked T waves consistent with **hyperkalemia** [ABIM code # 74]. Typical early changes of hyperkalemia include peaked T waves, shortened QT interval, and ST segment depression. Moderate hyperkalemia may cause bundle branch blocks, widening of the QRS complex, increases in the PR interval, and decreased amplitude of the P wave. If untreated, the P wave eventually disappears and the QRS morphology widens to resemble a sine wave. Ventricular fibrillation or asystole follows, leading to cardiac arrest.

2. Hyperkalemia can be treated with intravenous calcium to negate cardiac toxicity, glucose + insulin to increase intracellular uptake of potassium, and sodium bicarbonate to treat metabolic acidosis. Renal excretion can be increased with furosemide, and gastrointestinal excretion of potassium augmented by cation exchange resins such as sodium polystyrene sulfonate. Patients with severe hyperkalemia and renal dysfunction need emergent dialysis.

Case 13

13.1 Clinical Scenario

A 64-year-old male presents to your office for evaluation of chest discomfort. His past medical history is significant for hypertension, hyperlipidemia, rheumatic heart disease, and arthritis. On physical examination, he appears in moderate discomfort. His medications include atenolol and celebrex. He is afebrile, has a heart rate of 61 beats/minute, a respiratory rate of 18/minute, and a blood pressure of 147/79 mmHg. His cardiac examination reveals an elevated jugular venous pressure, an S4 gallop, a mid-diastolic rumble, and a prominent second heart sound in the pulmonary area. His lung examination is unremarkable. A qualitative test for cardiac troponin is positive.

13.2 Questions

1. What is the most likely diagnosis?

2. What does the ECG show?

3. What is the optimal treatment for this patient?

13.3 ECG Sample

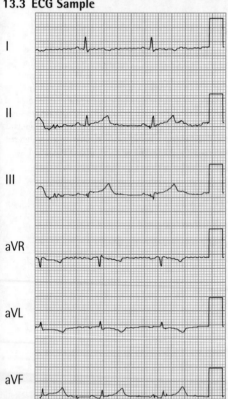

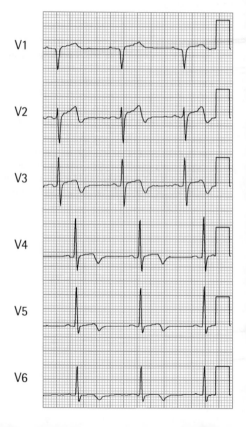

13.4 Answers

1. The most likely clinical diagnosis is an acute coronary syndrome.

2. The 12-lead ECG shows sinus rhythm [ABIM code # 7] and **ST segment and/or T wave suggesting myocardial ischemia** [ABIM code # 64]. The earliest signs of acute myocardial infarction may be subtle and include increased T wave amplitude over the affected area. T waves may become more prominent, symmetrical, and pointed ("hyperacute").
   These changes in T waves may only be present transiently after the onset of the ischemia and are usually followed by ST segment changes.

3. This patient should be treated with oxygen, nitrates, heparin, antiplatelet therapy, and statins. If he has persistent chest pain or elevation of cardiac biomarkers, coronary angiography may be indicated. If this evolves into an ST segment elevation myocardial infarction, he would be a candidate for thrombolysis or primary angioplasty.

Case 14

14.1 Clinical Scenario

A 63-year-old male presents to your office for routine evaluation. His past medical history is significant for hypertension and arthritis, and he informs you that he has previously undergone a cardiac procedure. On physical examination, he appears comfortable, without acute discomfort. He is afebrile, has a heart rate of 66 beats/minute, a respiratory rate of 14/minute, and a blood pressure of 136/66 mmHg. His cardiac examination reveals a short I/VI systolic murmur in the aortic area, and his lungs are clear to auscultation. You request a 12-lead ECG.

14.2 Questions

1. What does the ECG show?

2. What should you tell him about follow-up?

14.3 ECG Sample

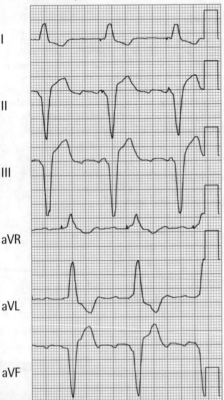

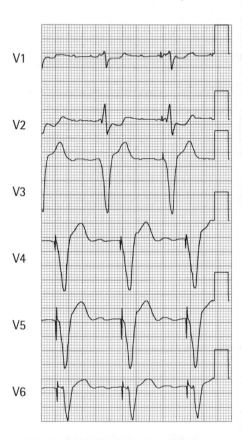

14.4 Answers

1. The 12-lead ECG shows sinus rhythm [ABIM code # 7] and a **ventricular demand pacemaker**, normally functioning [ABIM code # 91].

2. After implantation of a pacemaker, careful follow-up and continuity of care is mandatory. Frequency of follow-up is dictated by multiple factors, including other cardiovascular or medical problems managed by the physician involved, the age of the pacemaker, and the results of transtelephonic testing. Patients who are pacemaker dependent require more frequent clinical evaluations than those who are not. Follow-up evaluation usually includes assessment of battery status, pacing threshold and pulse width, sensing function, and lead integrity.

Case 15

15.1 Clinical Scenario

A 66-year-old male presents to your office with weakness and fatigue. His past medical history is significant for coronary artery disease, hypertension, and chronic obstructive pulmonary disease. His medications include digoxin, dyazide, and atorvastatin. On physical examination, he appears comfortable. He is afebrile, has a heart rate of 97 beats/minute, a respiratory rate of 14/minute, and a blood pressure of 129/74 mmHg. His cardiac examination reveals a Grade I/VI systolic murmur. You request a 12-lead ECG.

15.2 Questions

1. What does the ECG show?

2. What is the optimal treatment for this patient?

15.3 ECG Sample

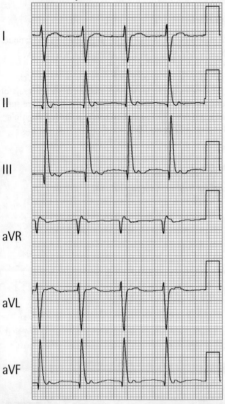

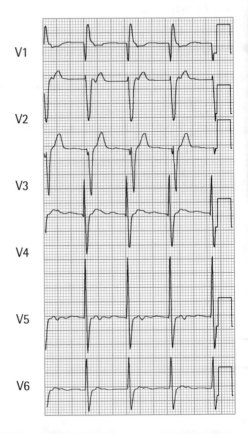

15.4 Answers

1. The 12-lead ECG shows accelerated **junctional rhythm** [ABIM code # 22], right-axis deviation [ABIM code # 38], and incomplete right bundle branch block [ABIM code # 44].

2. Accelerated junctional rhythm is an active junctional pacemaker rhythm caused usually by ischemia, drugs, and/or electrolyte abnormalities. Atrioventricular nodal junctional rhythms are generally well tolerated, but patients with coronary artery disease, those with significant co-morbidities, or elderly patients may not tolerate junctional rhythm well and may require treatment. Treatment strategy includes determination of the underlying cause and therapy directed to it. This patient had his digoxin discontinued, with resolution of the abnormal rhythm.

Case 16

16.1 Clinical Scenario

A 66-year-old male presents to your office for cardiac evaluation. His past medical history is significant for hypertension, coronary artery disease, and chronic obstructive pulmonary disease. His medications include amlodipine, thiazide diuretics, and nitrates. On physical examination, he appears comfortable and in no acute distress. He is afebrile, has a heart rate of 81 beats/minute, a respiratory rate of 14/minute, and a blood pressure of 119/65 mmHg. His cardiac examination reveals a soft first heart sound, without a gallop, rub, or murmur. You request a 12-lead ECG and a lipid profile.

16.2 Questions

1. What does the ECG show?

2. What is the optimal treatment for this patient?

16.3 ECG Sample

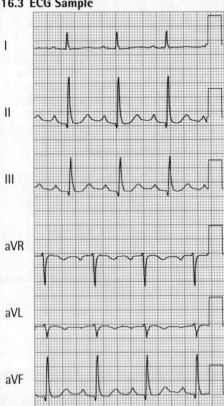

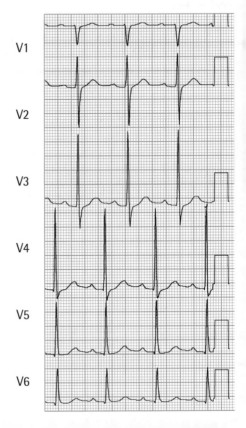

16.4 Answers

1. The 12-lead ECG shows sinus rhythm [ABIM code # 7], **primary atrioventricular (AV) block** [ABIM code # 29], and possible right atrial enlargement [ABIM code # 5].

2. Patients with first-degree AV block do not need any specific therapy but may be observed with follow-up ECGs over time to check for progression to higher-grade AV block.

Case 17

17.1 Clinical Scenario

A 79-year-old male is brought to the emergency room by his neighbors. After a blizzard over the weekend, the neighbors went to check on him and found him lethargic and drowsy. On physical examination, he appears cold, has a heart rate of 98 beats/minute, a respiratory rate of 16/minute, and a blood pressure of 103/72 mmHg. His cardiac examination is unremarkable. You request a 12-lead ECG.

17.2 Questions

1. What does the ECG show?

2. What is the optimal treatment for this patient?

17.3 ECG Sample

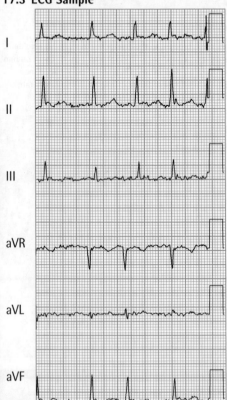

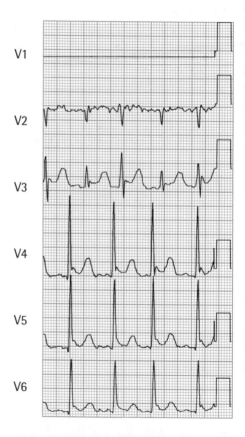

17.4 Answers

1. The 12-lead ECG shows normal atrial fibrillation [ABIM code # 19], motion/shivering artifact, prolonged Q-T interval [ABIM code # 68], and Osborne or J waves. All of these changes are consistent with **hypothermia** [ABIM code # 88].

2. Mildly hypothermic patients may be rewarmed with warm blankets and removal of cold or wet clothing. Profound hypothermia is a medical emergency and needs aggressive treatment. Therapies to maintain or restore cardiac perfusion and maximize oxygenation are indicated for a prolonged period of time, until the core temperature is at least 32-33°C.

Case 18

18.1 Clinical Scenario

A 19-year-old female presents to the emergency room with weakness, fatigue, and lethargy. She has had watery diarrhea for the past week, after a trip to Mexico. She is mildly febrile, has a heart rate of 70 beats/minute, respiratory rate of 16/minute, and a blood pressure of 89/65 mmHg. Her cardiac examination reveals normal heart sounds, without a gallop, rub, or murmur. You request a 12-lead ECG and a complete metabolic panel.

18.2 Questions

1. What does the ECG show?

2. What is the optimal treatment for this patient?

18.3 ECG Sample

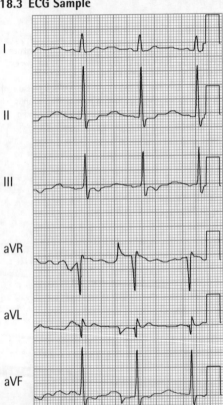

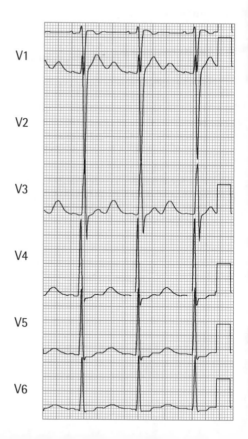

18.4 Answers

1. The 12-lead ECG shows sinus rhythm [ABIM code # 7], T wave
   flattening with inverted T waves, prominent U waves that appear as
   QT prolongation, and ST segment depression, all of which are consistent
   with **hypokalemia** [ABIM code # 75]. The ECG patterns seen in patients
   with hypokalemia range from mild T wave flattening to the appearance
   of prominent U waves, occasionally with ST segment depressions or
   T wave inversions. When the U wave is greater than the T wave, the
   potassium level is usually lower than 2.5 mEq/L. Hypokalemia may also
   cause atrial and ventricular arrhythmias. Her potassium level was
   2.4 mEq/L, consistent with severe hypokalemia.

2. Patients in whom severe hypokalemia is suspected should be placed on
   a cardiac monitor and an intravenous line placed. Potassium should be
   administered at 10–20 mEq/h IV via a peripheral or central line. Serum
   potassium is difficult to replenish if serum magnesium is also low, and a
   magnesium level should be checked in all patients with hypokalemia.

Case 19

19.1 Clinical Scenario

You are asked to see a 72-year-old man for an abnormal rhythm. He is admitted to the Neurology Department for evaluation of involuntary movements. His past medical history is significant for hypertension, benign prostatic hypertrophy, and dyslipidemia. On physical examination, he is afebrile, has a heart rate of 88 beats/minute, a respiratory rate of 16/minute, and a blood pressure of 123/72 mmHg. His cardiac examination is unremarkable. You request a 12-lead ECG.

19.2 Questions

1. What does the ECG show?

2. What is the optimal treatment for this patient?

19.3 ECG Sample

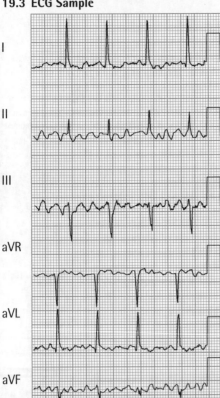

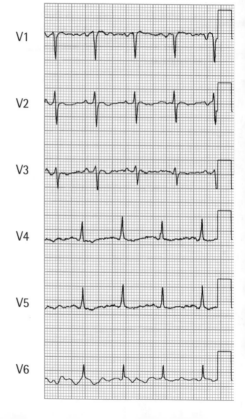

19.4 Answers

1. The 12-lead ECG shows normal sinus rhythm [ABIM code # 7] and muscle tremor **artifact** mimicking atrial fibrillation [ABIM code # 4].

2. No treatment is indicated in this patient, except reassurance about the abnormal ECG.

Case 20

20.1 Clinical Scenario

A 33-year-old male presents to your office with a history of episodic palpitations and lightheadedness. On physical examination, he is comfortable, afebrile, has a heart rate of 60 beats/minute, and a blood pressure of 128/65 mmHg. You request a 12-lead ECG.

20.2 Questions

1. What does the ECG show?

2. How should he be treated?

20.3 ECG Sample

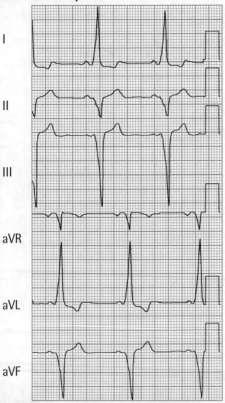

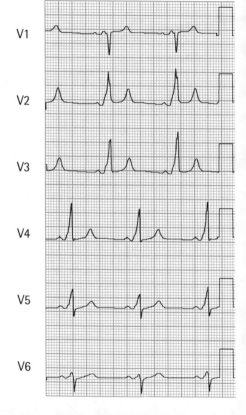

20.4 Answers

1. The 12-lead ECG shows a shortened PR interval, a widened QRS complex, and a delta wave consistent with **Wolff–Parkinson–White (WPW) pattern** [ABIM code # 34].

2. WPW syndrome is the most common pre-excitation syndrome with an accessory atrioventricular (AV) pathway otherwise known as the Kent bundle. Conduction through a Kent bundle can be anterograde, retrograde, or both. Normal individuals are protected from exceptionally high heart rates during atrial fibrillation by the relatively long refractory period of the AV node. In patients with WPW, however, the accessory pathway often has a much shorter anterograde refractory period, allowing for much faster transmission of impulses and correspondingly higher heart rates and potential degeneration into ventricular fibrillation. If atrial fibrillation were to be treated in the conventional manner by drugs that prolong the refractory period of the AV node (e.g. calcium channel blockers, beta-blockers, digoxin), the rate of transmission through the accessory pathway may increase, with a corresponding increase in ventricular rate. This may cause the arrhythmia to deteriorate into ventricular fibrillation. Procainamide (17 mg/kg IV infusion, not to exceed 50 mg/minute) blocks the accessory pathway and is the preferred agent. Prompt cardioversion of patients with WPW and atrial fibrillation presenting with hypotension is indicated. Definitive therapy is ablation of the accessory pathway, which may be considered in this patient, based on the frequency of episodes of tachyarrhythmia.

Case 21

21.1 Clinical Scenario

A 63-year-old male presents to the emergency room with chest discomfort and fatigue. He gives a history of chest heaviness and generalized weakness for the past several days. His past medical history is significant for hypertension and coronary artery disease. On physical examination, he appears lethargic but in no acute distress. He is afebrile, has a heart rate of 52 beats/minute, a respiratory rate of 14/minute, and a blood pressure of 108/54 mmHg. His cardiac examination reveals changing intensity of the first heart sound and he has a few crackles on lung examination. You request a 12-lead ECG.

21.2 Questions

1. What does the ECG show?

2. What is the optimal treatment for this patient?

21.3 ECG Sample

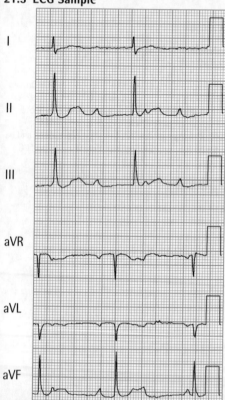

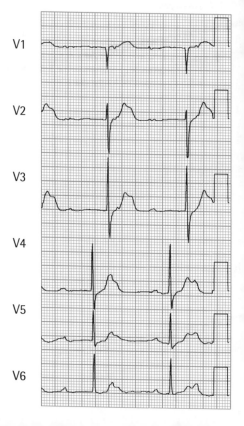

21.4 Answers

1. The 12-lead ECG shows sinus rhythm [ABIM code # 7], **AV dissociation** [ABIM code # 35], and junctional escape complexes [ABIM code # 21].

2. This patient with chest heaviness and atrioventricular dissociation most likely has an acute coronary syndrome and should be investigated and treated appropriately for this. Once ischemia resolves, his rhythm may revert back to normal.

Case 22

22.1 Clinical Scenario

A 59-year-old male presents to your office for follow-up evaluation. His past medical history is significant for dilated non-ischemic cardiomyopathy, congestive heart failure, and renal insufficiency. His medications include digoxin, carvedilol, and losartan. On physical examination, he is comfortable, afebrile, has a heart rate of 93 beats/minute, and a blood pressure of 133/81 mmHg. You request a 12-lead ECG.

22.2 Questions

1. What does the ECG show?

2. How should he be treated?

22.3 ECG Sample

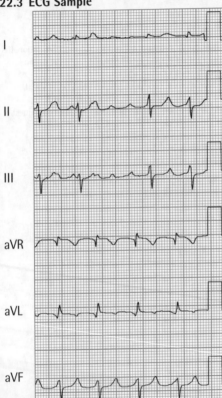

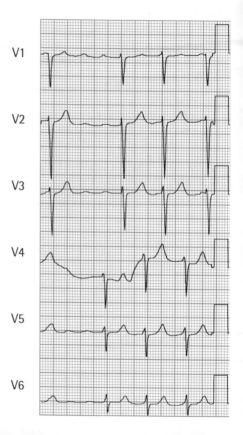

22.4 Answers

1. The 12-lead ECG shows **paroxysmal atrial tachycardia with variable block** [ABIM code # 15] consistent with **digoxin toxicity** [ABIM code # 71].

2. Digoxin toxicity is an important cause of atrial tachycardia, with triggered activity as the underlying mechanism. Atrial tachycardia due to digitalis intoxication often manifests with atrioventricular conduction block and/or ventricular arrhythmias. Recognizing this at an early stage is important because it may be a harbinger of more malignant ventricular arrhythmias. Treatment includes prompt discontinuation of digoxin and correction of electrolyte disturbances. The administration of antidigoxin antibodies is usually indicated in patients with high-grade conduction block, severe bradycardia, and ventricular arrhythmias. Electrical cardioversion of atrial dysrhythmias is usually not indicated because it may precipitate a ventricular tachyarrhythmia.

Case 23

23.1 Clinical Scenario

A 32-year-old female presents to your office for routine evaluation. Her past medical history is significant for episodes of palpitations. On physical examination, she appears comfortable and in no acute distress. She is afebrile, has a heart rate of 120 beats/minute, a respiratory rate of 14/minute, and a blood pressure of 107/66 mmHg. Her cardiac examination reveals a loud first heart sound with a wide split and a Grade II/IV diastolic murmur in the tricuspid area that increases with inspiration.

23.2 Questions

1. What is the most likely diagnosis?

2. What does the ECG show?

3. What is the optimal treatment for this patient?

23.3 ECG Sample

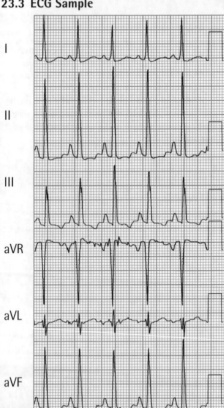

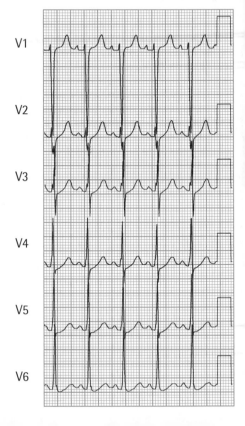

23.4 Answers

1. The most likely clinical diagnosis is tricuspid stenosis.

2. The 12-lead ECG shows **sinus tachycardia** [ABIM code # 10], with tall
    P waves in lead II, III, and aVF consistent with right atrial enlargement
    [ABIM code # 5].

3. Tricuspid stenosis is a narrowing of the tricuspid valve that increases
    resistance to blood flow from the right atrium to the right ventricle.
    Symptoms are usually mild and include palpitations, cold skin, and
    fatigue. Palpitations can be effectively treated with beta-blockers,
    which would also increase the time for right ventricular filling by
    prolonging diastole. Definitive therapy includes balloon valvuloplasty or
    valve surgery.

Case 24

24.1 Clinical Scenario

A 44-year-old female is referred to you by her primary care physician for an irregular pulse. Her past medical history is unremarkable. On physical examination, she appears comfortable and in no acute distress. She is afebrile, has a heart rate of 66 beats/minute, a respiratory rate of 14/minute, and a blood pressure of 107/66 mmHg. Her cardiac examination reveals a soft, Grade I/VI systolic murmur in the mitral area. You request a 12-lead ECG.

24.2 Questions

1. What does the ECG show?

2. What is the optimal treatment for this patient?

24.3 ECG Sample

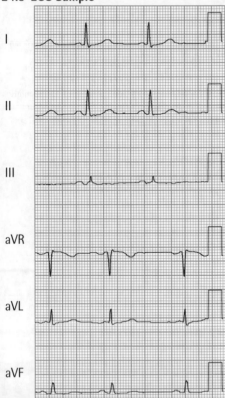

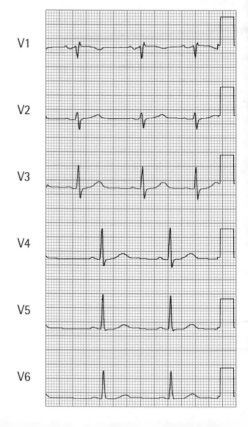

24.4 Answers

1. The 12-lead ECG shows **sinus arrhythmia** [ABIM code # 8], but is otherwise normal [ABIM code # 1].

2. Sinus arrhythmia refers to the normal cyclical changes in the timing of the heart rate and does not require specific therapy. The patient needs to be reassured.

Case 25

25.1 Clinical Scenario

A 71-year-old male presents to your office for routine evaluation. His past medical history is significant for hypertension and arthritis, and he informs you that he has previously undergone a cardiac procedure. On physical examination, he appears comfortable, without acute discomfort. He is afebrile, has a heart rate of 66 beats/minute, a respiratory rate of 14/minute, and a blood pressure of 136/66 mmHg. His cardiac examination reveals a short I/VI systolic murmur in the aortic area, and his lungs are clear to auscultation. You request a 12-lead ECG.

25.2 Questions

1. What does the ECG show?

2. What should you tell him about follow-up?

25.3 ECG Sample

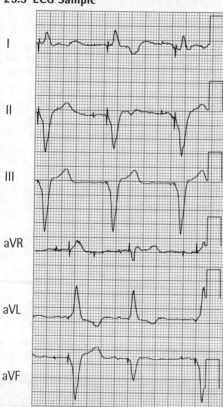

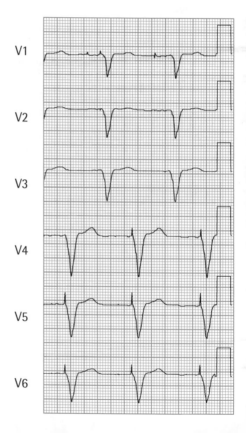

25.4 Answers

1. The 12-lead ECG shows a **dual–chamber pacemaker**, which is functioning normally [ABIM code # 92].

2. After implantation of a pacemaker, careful follow-up and continuity of care is mandatory. Frequency of follow-up is dictated by multiple factors, including other cardiovascular or medical problems managed by the physician involved, the age of the pacemaker, and the results of transtelephonic testing. Patients who are pacemaker dependent require more frequent clinical evaluations than those who are not. Follow-up evaluation usually includes assessment of battery status, pacing threshold and pulse width, sensing function, and lead integrity.

Case 26

26.1 Clinical Scenario

A 63-year-old female presents to your office for evaluation of chronic dyspnea, which has worsened in the past week. She has a 40-pack-year smoking history and her past medical history is significant for hypertension. On physical examination, she appears tachypneic and has some audible wheezing. She is afebrile, has a heart rate of 130 beats/minute, a respiratory rate of 22/minute, and a blood pressure of 137/66 mmHg. Her cardiac examination reveals an elevated jugular venous pressure and an S4 gallop. Her lung examination reveals bilateral rhonchi.

26.2 Questions

1. What does the ECG show?

2. What is the optimal treatment for this patient?

26.3 ECG Sample

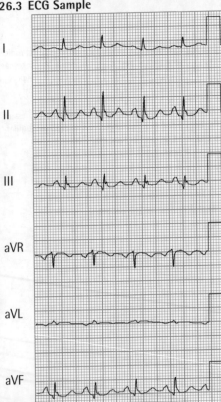

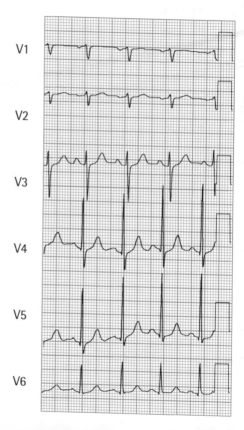

26.4 Answers

1. The 12-lead ECG shows sinus tachycardia [ABIM code # 10], with tall P
   waves in lead II, III, and aVF consistent with **right atrial enlargement**
   [ABIM code # 5].

2. Acute exacerbations of chronic obstructive pulmonary disease result in
   significant morbidity and mortality, and exacerbations requiring
   hospital admission are associated with an in-hospital mortality rate of
   3-4%. Early aggressive treatment with bronchodilators, corticosteroids,
   and antibiotics in appropriate patients are indicated. Indications for
   mechanical ventilation include labored breathing with respiratory rates
   of more than 30 breaths per minute, moderate to severe respiratory
   acidosis, decreased level of consciousness, and respiratory arrest.

Case 27

27.1 Clinical Scenario

You are asked to see a 66-year-old male for an abnormal rhythm two days after coronary bypass surgery. His medications include atenolol, lipitor, and losartan. On physical examination, he is in mild distress, is afebrile, has a heart rate of 143 beats/minute, and a blood pressure of 113/81 mmHg. You request a 12-lead ECG.

27.2 Questions

1. What does the ECG show?

2. How should he be treated?

27.3 ECG Sample

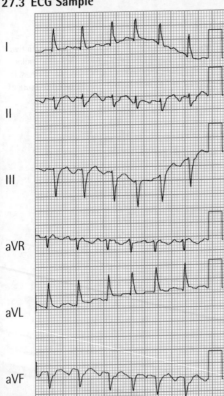

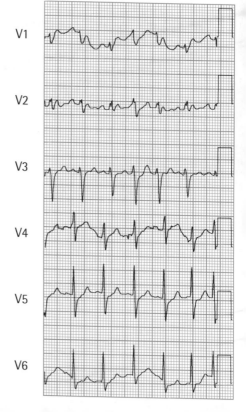

27.4 Answers

1. The 12-lead ECG shows **atrial tachycardia with variable block** [ABIM code # 15], left anterior fascicular block [ABIM code # 45], and non-specific ST segment and/or T wave abnormalities [ABIM code # 63].

2. Treatment is directed at the underlying cardiopulmonary process or metabolic abnormality. Specific antiarrhythmic therapy is not commonly indicated, and the value of such therapy is unproven. Beta-blockers have been shown to be effective in controlling heart rate and may sometimes convert the abnormal rhythm to normal sinus rhythm.

Case 28

28.1 Clinical Scenario

A 39-year-old female presents for evaluation of occasional palpitations and dyspnea on severe exertion. On physical examination, she is afebrile, has a heart rate of 80 beats/minute, and a blood pressure of 113/81 mmHg. You request a 12-lead ECG.

28.2 Questions

1. What does the ECG show?

2. What is the next step?

28.3 ECG Sample

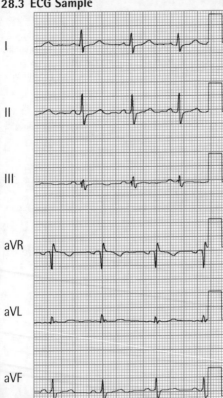

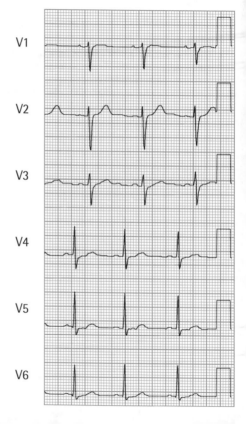

28.4 Answers

1. The 12-lead ECG shows sinus rhythm [ABIM code # 7], and is a **normal ECG** [ABIM code # 1].

2. No treatment is indicated based on the ECG. She may need further cardiopulmonary testing if clinically indicated, but dyspnea on severe exertion may be related to deconditioning. If she continues to have palpitations, a Holter monitor or an event recorder would be useful.

Case 29

29.1 Clinical Scenario

You are asked to see a 67-year-old male for an abnormal rhythm. He underwent an aortobifemoral bypass three days ago and has been complaining of chest pain for the past three hours. On physical examination, he has a faint pulse, with a blood pressure of 66/34 mmHg. You request a 12-lead ECG.

29.2 Questions

1. What does the ECG show?

2. How should this patient be treated?

29.3 ECG Sample

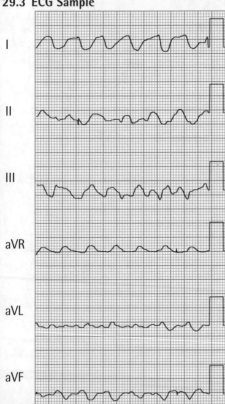

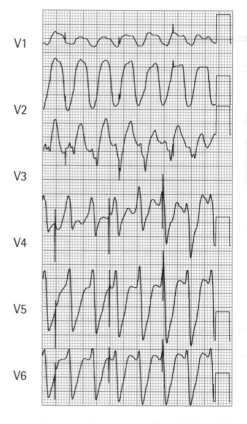

29.4 Answers

1. The ECG shows **ventricular tachycardia (VT)** [ABIM code # 25]. Typical findings for VT may include the absence of RS complexes in the precordial ECG leads (V1-V6), RS duration greater than 100 milliseconds in any precordial lead, and atrioventricular (AV) dissociation.
   The presence of capture or fusion beats may also be helpful.

   ECG criteria for VT include:
   • Atrioventricular dissociation
   • QRS axis between minus 90 degrees and plus or minus 180 degrees
   • Positive QRS concordance (positive QRS V1-V6)
   • QRS duration ≥ 140 milliseconds with a right bundle branch block pattern and ≥ 160 milliseconds with a left bundle branch block pattern
   • Combination of a left bundle branch block pattern and right-axis deviation
   • Monophasic or biphasic QRS complex with a right bundle branch block pattern and a slurred or prolonged S wave in V1 with left bundle branch block morphology
   • **Fusion beats.** Fusion beats indicate the activation of the ventricle from two foci, implying that one is of ventricular origin. When two impulses invade the ventricle simultaneously, each impulse activates that part of the ventricle, and the resulting QRS complex has a configuration that is between that of a QRS complex of the ectopic beat and the QRS complex of a sinus beat.

- **Capture beats.** A capture beat is the momentary activation of the ventricles by the sinus impulse during AV dissociation. During VT, the slower sinus impulse cannot be conducted antegradely to the ventricles. The sinus impulse may occasionally reach the AV node when it is no longer refractory, and is able to penetrate and capture the ventricles, resulting in a capture beat. A capture beat resembles the QRS complex of a normal sinus impulse and is preceded by a P wave. The presence of fusion beats and capture beats provides the best support for the diagnosis of VT, although they are not very commonly seen.

2. The management of VT depends upon the hemodynamic consequences of the dysrhythmia. VT associated with loss of consciousness, hypotension, or pulmonary edema is a medical emergency requiring immediate cardioversion. This is done with a 200–360 J monophasic shock or an equivalent biphasic energy dose. When the patient is stable, a trial of medical therapy may be considered. If left ventricular function is impaired, amiodarone or lidocaine is favored over procainamide because of the potential of the latter to exacerbate heart failure. If medical therapy is unsuccessful, synchronized cardioversion following conscious sedation should be performed. This person with hypotension should be cardioverted immediately. He should also be evaluated for post-operative myocardial ischemia or infarction.

ECG pocket

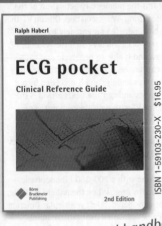

Ralph Haberl

ECG pocket

Clinical Reference Guide

Börm Bruckmeier Publishing

2nd Edition

ISBN 1-59103-230-X $16.95

- Handy reference for identifying common ECG findings

- Top-quality collection of numerous digital 12-lead ECGs

- Provides a quick reference section and a standardized ECG evaluation sheet

- For students, residents and all other health care professionals

more pocket-sized handbooks

English - Spanish / Spanish - English

Medical Spanish pocket plus

Börm Bruckmeier Publishing

ISBN 1-59103-213-X $22.95

Spanish for Medical Professionals

Medical Spanish pocket

Börm Bruckmeier Publishing

2nd Edition

ISBN 1-59103-232-6 $16.95

Spanish for Medical Professionals

Medical Spanish Dictionary pocket

Börm Bruckmeier Publishing

2nd Edition

ISBN 1-59103-231-8 $16.95

www.media4u.com

Case 30

30.1 Clinical Scenario

A 53-year-old male presents to the emergency department with substernal chest discomfort for the past 30 minutes. His past medical history is significant for hypertension, hyperlipidemia, and diabetes mellitus. On physical examination, he appears diaphoretic and in significant chest discomfort. He is afebrile, has a heart rate of 92 beats/minute, a respiratory rate of 20/minute, and a blood pressure of 101/66 mmHg. His cardiac examination reveals an elevated jugular venous pressure, an S4 gallop, and a Grade II/VI apical systolic murmur. His lungs are clear to auscultation.

30.2 Questions

1. What is the most likely diagnosis?

2. What should be the next diagnostic test?

3. What does the ECG show?

4. What is the optimal treatment for this patient?

30.3 ECG Sample

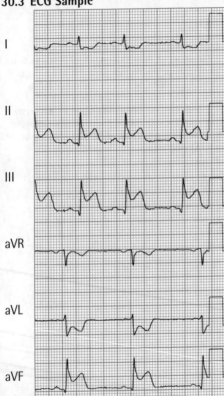

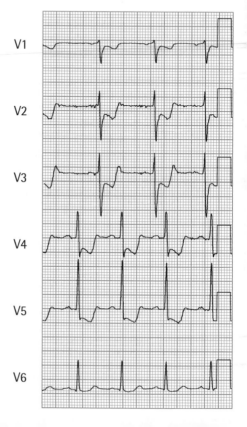

30.4 Answers

1. The most likely clinical diagnosis is an acute coronary syndrome, which may include unstable angina, non-ST segment elevation myocardial infarction [NSTEMI] and ST segment elevation myocardial infarction [STEMI].

2. The next diagnostic test should include an ECG within 10 minutes of clinical presentation. A 12-lead ECG should be performed and shown to an experienced emergency physician within 10 minutes of emergency room arrival for all patients with chest discomfort (or anginal equivalent) or other symptoms suggestive of STEMI.
   [ACC/AHA Guidelines for the Management of Patients With ST-Elevation Myocardial Infarction-Executive Summary].

3. The 12-lead ECG shows normal sinus rhythm [ABIM code # 7] and **ST segment and/or T wave abnormalities suggesting myocardial injury** [ABIM code # 65]. The ECG also shows ST segment and/or T wave abnormalities suggestive of anterolateral myocardial ischemia [ABIM code # 64].

4. For patients with ST segment elevation on the 12-lead ECG, reperfusion therapy should be initiated as soon as possible, without waiting for cardiac biomarker results. This patient should preferably be sent to the cardiac catheterization laboratory for primary angioplasty; if such facilities are not available and the likely transfer time is more than 60 minutes, fibrinolytics should be administered. If immediately available, primary percutaneous intervention (PCI) should be performed in patients with STEMI (including true posterior myocardial infarction) or myocardial infarction with new or presumably new left bundle branch block who can undergo PCI of the infarct artery within 12 hours of symptom onset, if performed in a timely fashion (balloon inflation within 90 minutes of presentation) by persons skilled in the procedure.

Case 31

31.1 Clinical Scenario

A 69-year-old male presents to the emergency room with substernal chest discomfort for the past three hours. His past medical history is significant for hypertension, hyperlipidemia, and prior stroke.

On physical examination, he appears diaphoretic and in moderate discomfort. He is afebrile, has a heart rate of 96 beats/minute, a respiratory rate of 20/minute, and a blood pressure of 154/96 mmHg. His cardiac examination reveals a mildly elevated jugular venous pressure, an S4 gallop, and a soft, Grade I/VI systolic murmur. His lung examination reveals a few bibasilar rales. On routine blood work, his blood glucose is 144 mg/dL, hemoglobin is 14.2 g/dL, platelet count is 328×10^9/L, and creatinine is 1.2 mg/dL.

31.2 Questions

1. What is the most likely diagnosis?

2. What should be the next diagnostic test?

3. What does the ECG show?

4. What is the optimal treatment for this patient?

31.3 ECG Sample

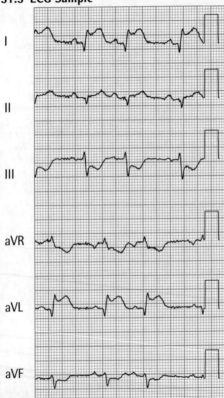

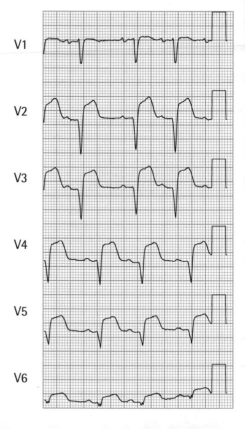

31.4 Answers

1. The most likely clinical diagnosis is an acute coronary syndrome, which may include unstable angina, non-ST segment elevation myocardial infarction [NSTEMI] or ST segment elevation myocardial infarction [STEMI].

2. The next diagnostic test should include an ECG within 10 minutes of clinical presentation. A 12-lead ECG should be performed and shown to an experienced emergency physician within 10 minutes of emergency room arrival for all patients with chest discomfort (or anginal equivalent) or other symptoms suggestive of STEMI. [ACC/AHA Guidelines for the Management of Patients With ST-Elevation Myocardial Infarction-Executive Summary].

3. The 12-lead ECG shows normal sinus rhythm [ABIM code # 7], with sinus arrhythmia [ABIM code # 8], an acute ST segment elevation **anterolateral myocardial infarction**, with ST segment elevation in leads V2-V6, I, and aVL [ABIM code # 51], and ST segment and/or T wave abnormalities suggesting myocardial injury [ABIM code # 65]. If only ST segment elevation is present, without significant Q waves, the ECG should be coded as myocardial injury and not as myocardial infarction.

4. For patients with ST segment elevation on the 12-lead ECG, reperfusion therapy should be initiated as soon as possible, without waiting for cardiac biomarker results. This patient should preferably be sent to the cardiac catheterization laboratory for primary angioplasty; if such facilities are not available and the likely transfer time is more than 60 minutes, fibrinolytics should be administered. If immediately available, primary percutaneous intervention (PCI) should be performed in patients with STEMI (including true posterior myocardial infarction) or myocardial infarctionwith new or presumably new left bundle branch block who can undergo PCI of the infarct artery within 12 hours of symptom onset, if performed in a timely fashion (balloon inflation within 90 minutes of presentation) by persons skilled in the procedure.

Case 32

32.1 Clinical Scenario

A 73-year-old female presents to the emergency department with substernal chest discomfort for the past hour. Her past medical history is significant for hypertension, hyperlipidemia, and diet-controlled diabetes mellitus. On physical examination, she appears diaphoretic and in significant discomfort. She is afebrile, has a heart rate of 98 beats/minute, a respiratory rate of 20/minute, and a blood pressure of 98/66 mmHg. Her cardiac examination reveals an elevated jugular venous pressure, an S4 gallop, and a Grade II/VI apical systolic murmur. Her lungs are clear to auscultation. On routine blood work, her blood glucose is 167 mg/dL, hemoglobin is 13.3 g/dL, platelet count is 268×10^9/L, and creatinine is 1.3 mg/dL.

32.2 Questions

1. What is the most likely diagnosis?

2. What should be the next diagnostic test?

3. What does the ECG show?

4. What is the optimal treatment for this patient?

32.3 ECG Sample

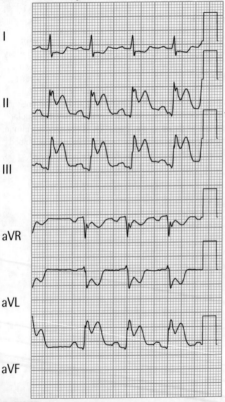

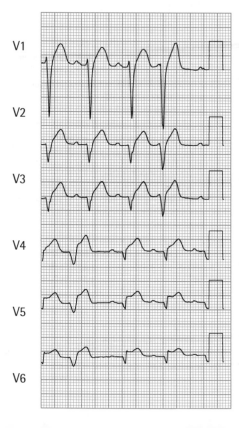

32.4 Answers

1. The most likely clinical diagnosis is an acute coronary syndrome, which may include unstable angina, NSTEMI and STEMI.

2. The next diagnostic test should include an ECG within 10 minutes of clinical presentation. A 12-lead ECG should be performed and shown to an experienced emergency physician within 10 minutes of emergency room arrival for all patients with chest discomfort (or anginal equivalent) or other symptoms suggestive of STEMI.
    [ACC/AHA Guidelines for the Management of Patients With ST-Elevation Myocardial Infarction-Executive Summary].

3. The 12-lead ECG shows normal sinus rhythm [ABIM code # 7], with premature ventricular complexes [ABIM code # 23], an acute ST segment elevation **inferior myocardial infarction**, with ST segment elevation in leads II, III, and aVF [ABIM code # 57], acute lateral wall myocardial infarction with ST segment elevation in leads V4–V6 [ABIM code # 55], and ST segment and/or T wave abnormalities suggesting myocardial injury [ABIM code # 65]. The ECG also shows a non-specific intraventricular conduction delay [ABIM code # 49].

4. For patients with ST segment elevation on the 12-lead ECG, reperfusion therapy should be initiated as soon as possible, without waiting for cardiac biomarker results. This patient should preferably be sent to the cardiac catheterization laboratory for primary angioplasty; if such facilities are not available and the likely transfer time is more than 60 minutes, fibrinolytics should be administered. If immediately available, primary percutaneous intervention (PCI) should be performed in patients with STEMI (including true posterior myocardial infarction) or myocardial infarction with new or presumably new left bundle branch block who can undergo PCI of the infarct artery within 12 hours of symptom onset, if performed in a timely fashion (balloon inflation within 90 minutes of presentation) by persons skilled in the procedure.

Clinical Scenario 143

Case 33

33.1 Clinical Scenario

A 55-year-old male presents to the emergency department with substernal chest discomfort for the past hour. His past medical history is significant for hypertension, hyperlipidemia, and peptic ulcer disease. On physical examination, he appears diaphoretic and in moderate discomfort. He is afebrile, has a heart rate of 48 beats/minute, a respiratory rate of 20/minute, and a blood pressure of 88/56 mmHg. His cardiac examination reveals an elevated jugular venous pressure and an S4 gallop. His lungs are clear to auscultation. On routine blood work, his blood glucose is 134 mg/dL, hemoglobin is 12.8 g/dL, platelet count is 271×10^9/L, and creatinine is 1.1 mg/dL.

33.2 Questions

1. What is the most likely diagnosis?

2. What should be the next diagnostic test?

3. What does the ECG show?

4. What is the optimal treatment for this patient?

33.3 ECG Sample

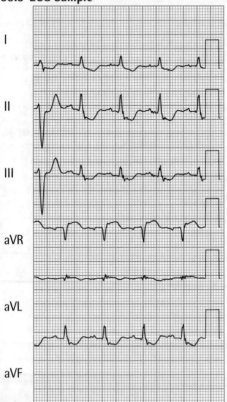

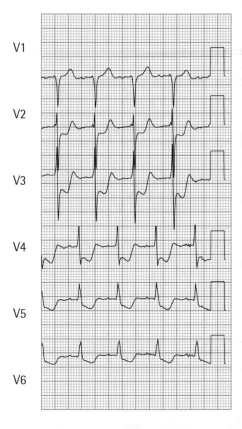

33.4 Answers

1. The most likely clinical diagnosis is an acute coronary syndrome, which may include unstable angina, NSTEMI and STEMI.

2. The next diagnostic test should include an ECG within 10 minutes of clinical presentation. A 12-lead ECG should be performed and shown to an experienced emergency physician within 10 minutes of emergency room arrival for all patients with chest discomfort (or anginal equivalent) or other symptoms suggestive of STEMI.
   [ACC/AHA Guidelines for the Management of Patients With ST-Elevation Myocardial Infarction-Executive Summary].

3. The 12-lead ECG shows sinus tachycardia [ABIM code # 10] and acute **posterior wall myocardial infarction**, with ST segment depression in leads V1–V4 [ABIM code # 59] and ST segment and/or T wave abnormalities suggesting myocardial injury [ABIM code # 65]. The ECG does not have a lead that directly faces the posterior wall of the heart. However, abnormalities of depolarization will cause reciprocal or mirror changes in the anterior leads (i.e. V1, V2, and V3, of which V2 is the most important).

4. For patients with ST segment elevation on the 12-lead ECG, or ST segment changes consistent with true posterior wall MI, reperfusion therapy should be initiated as soon as possible, without waiting for cardiac biomarker results. This patient should preferably be sent to the cardiac catheterization laboratory for primary angioplasty; if such facilities are not available and likely transfer time is more than 60 minutes, fibrinolytics should be administered. If immediately available, primary percutaneous intervention (PCI) should be performed in patients with STEMI (including true posterior MI) or MI with new or presumably new LBBBk who can undergo PCI of the infarct artery within 12 hours of symptom onset, if performed in a timely fashion (balloon inflation within 90 minutes of presentation) by persons skilled in the procedure.

Case 34

34.1 Clinical Scenario

A 67-year-old male presents to the emergency department with left arm discomfort for the last 30 minutes. His past medical history is significant for hypertension, hyperlipidemia, and diet controlled diabetes mellitus. On physical examination, he appears in moderate discomfort. He is afebrile, has a heart rate of 48/min, respiratory rate of 18/min and a blood pressure of 78/56 mmHg. His cardiac examination reveals an elevated jugular venous pressure and cardiac examination reveals a S4 gallop. His lungs are clear to auscultation.

34.2 Questions

1. What is the most likely diagnosis?

2. What should be the next diagnostic test?

3. What does the ECG show?

4. How should this patient be optimally treated and does he need a pacemaker?

34.3 ECG Sample

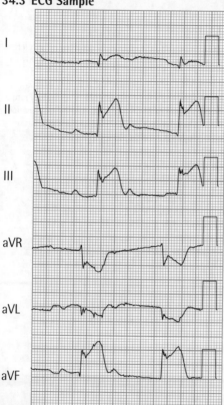

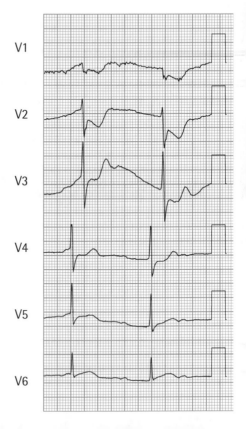

34.4 Answers

1. The most likely clinical diagnosis is an acute coronary syndrome which may include unstable angina, non ST-elevation myocardial infarction [NSTEMI] and ST-elevation myocardial infarction [STEMI].

2. The next diagnostic test should include an ECG within 10 minutes of clinical presentation. A 12-lead ECG should be performed and shown to an experienced emergency physician within 10 minutes of ED arrival for all patients with chest discomfort (or anginal equivalent) or other symptoms suggestive of STEMI. [ACC/AHA Guidelines for the Management of Patients With ST-Elevation Myocardial Infarction-Executive Summary].

3. The 12-lead ECG shows sinus rhythm [ABIM code # 7], ST and/or T wave abnormalities suggesting myocardial injury of the inferior wall [ABIM code # 65] and **complete heart block** [ABIM code # 33]. Since Q waves are not yet present in the inferior leads, the ECG should be coded as myocardial injury and not as an infarct.

4. For patients with ST elevation on the 12-lead ECG reperfusion therapy should be initiated as soon as possible and one should not wait for cardiac biomarker results. This patient should preferably be sent to the cardiac catheterization laboratory for primary angioplasty and if such facilities are not available and likely transfer time is more than 60 minutes fibrinolytics should be administered. If immediately available, primary PCI should be performed in patients with STEMI (including true posterior MI) or MI with new or presumably new LBBB who can undergo PCI of the infarct artery within 12 hours of symptom onset. Insertion of a temporary pacemaker should be considered in this patient with complete heart block and hypotension. If his AV node recovers from ischemia he may not need a permanent pacemaker.

Case 35

35.1 Clinical Scenario

A 63-year-old male presents to your office with exertional chest discomfort. His past medical history is significant for hypertension and arthritis. On physical examination, he appears comfortable, without acute discomfort. He is afebrile, has a heart rate of 86 beats/minute, a respiratory rate of 14/minute, and a blood pressure of 136/66 mmHg. His cardiac examination reveals an S4 gallop and a late peaking IV/VI ejection systolic murmur in the aortic area His lungs are clear to auscultation.

35.2 Questions

1. What is the most likely diagnosis?

2. What should be the next diagnostic test?

3. What does the ECG show?

4. What is the optimal treatment for this patient?

35.3 ECG Sample

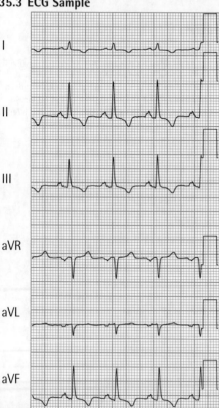

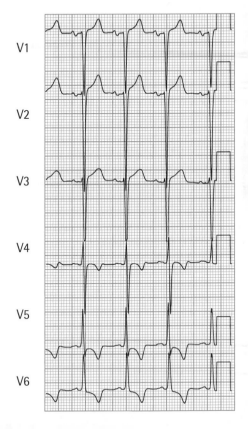

35.4 Answers

1. The most likely clinical diagnosis is acute aortic stenosis.

2. The next diagnostic test should be an echocardiogram to evaluate his aortic valve and left ventricular function.

3. The 12-lead ECG shows sinus rhythm [ABIM code # 7], **left ventricular hypertrophy (LVH)** [ABIM code # 40], and ST segment and/or T wave changes secondary to hypertrophy [ABIM code # 67].

   ECG criteria for LVH include:
   - R in aVL >9 mm (females) and >11 mm (males)
   - R in aVL + S in V3 > 20 mm (females), and > 25 mm (males)

   Sokolow-Lyon criteria:
   S in V1 + R in V5 or in V6 (whichever is taller) >35 mm

   Romhilt-Estes criteria:
   Points are given for QRS voltage, the presence of left atrial enlargement, and typical repolarization abnormalities. The combination of left atrial enlargement and typical repolarization abnormalities (score >5 points) will suffice for the diagnosis of LVH, even when voltage criteria are not met.

   Cornell criteria:
   - In males, S in V3 + R in aVL >28 mm
   - In females, S in V3 + R aVL >20 mm

4. Severe aortic stenosis was confirmed in this patient with an echocardiogram, showing an aortic valve area of 0.8 cm^2. Because the patient has symptomatic aortic stenosis, he would be a candidate for aortic valve surgery.

Case 36

36.1 Clinical Scenario

A 47-year-old male presents to your office for evaluation of shortness of breath. He has a 30-pack-year smoking history and his past medical history is significant for hypertension. On physical examination, he appears tachypneic and has audible wheezing. He is afebrile, has a heart rate of 130 beats/minute, a respiratory rate of 22/minute, and a blood pressure of 127/69 mmHg. His cardiac examination reveals an elevated jugular venous pressure and an S4 gallop. His lung examination reveals bilateral rhonchi.

36.2 Questions

1. What is the most likely diagnosis?

2. What does the ECG show?

3. What is the optimal treatment for this patient?

36.3 ECG Sample

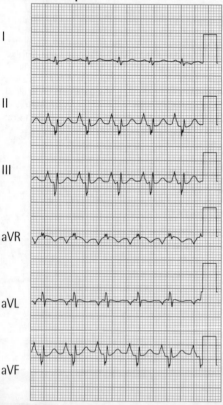

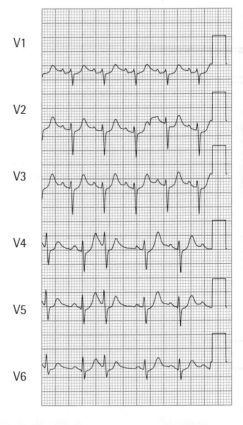

36.4 Answers

1. The most likely clinical diagnosis is chronic obstructive pulmonary disease (COPD) with an acute exacerbation.

2. The 12-lead ECG shows sinus tachycardia [ABIM code # 10], with tall P waves in leads II, III, and aVF consistent with **right atrial enlargement** [ABIM code # 5], and atrial premature complexes [ABIM code # 13]. This ECG demonstrates a constellation of findings suggestive of COPD, namely, sinus tachycardia, P pulmonale, and poor R wave progression in chest leads consistent with clockwise rotation.

3. Acute exacerbations of COPD result in significant morbidity and mortality, and exacerbations requiring hospital admission are associated with an in-hospital mortality rate of 3-4%. Early aggressive treatment with bronchodilators, corticosteroids, and antibiotics in appropriate patients are indicated. Indications for mechanical ventilation include labored breathing with respiratory rates of more than 30 breaths per minute, moderate to severe respiratory acidosis, decreased level of consciousness, and respiratory arrest.

Case 37

37.1 Clinical Scenario

A 57-year-old male presents to your office for evaluation of chest discomfort. His past medical history is significant for hypertension, hyperlipidemia, rheumatic heart disease, and arthritis. On physical examination, he appears in moderate discomfort. His medications include atenolol and celebrex. He is afebrile, has a heart rate of 68 beats/minute, a respiratory rate of 18/minute, and a blood pressure of 157/79 mmHg. His cardiac examination reveals an elevated jugular venous pressure, an S4 gallop, a mid-diastolic rumble, and a prominent second heart sound in the pulmonary area. His lung examination is unremarkable.

37.2 Questions

1. What is the most likely diagnosis?

2. What does the ECG show?

3. What is the optimal treatment for this patient?

37.3 ECG Sample

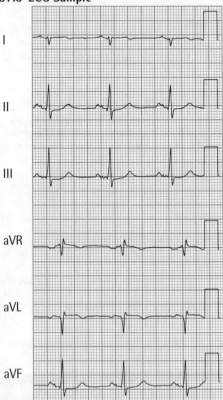

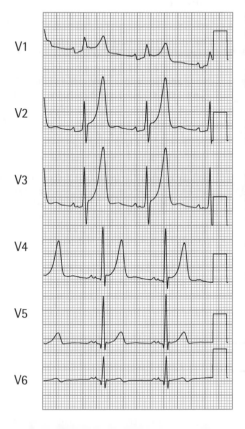

37.4 Answers

1. The most likely clinical diagnosis is an acute coronary syndrome.

2. The 12-lead ECG shows sinus rhythm [ABIM code # 7], with wide
   P waves in leads II, III, and aVF consistent with left atrial enlargement
   [ABIM code # 6], tall R waves in leads V1 and V2 consistent with right
   ventricular hypertrophy [ABIM code # 41], and **ST segment and /or
   T wave suggesting myocardial ischemia** [ABIM code 64]. The earliest
   signs of acute myocardial infarction may be subtle and include
   increased T wave amplitude over the affected area. T waves may become
   more prominent, symmetrical, and pointed ("hyperacute").
   These changes in T waves may only be present transiently after the
   onset of the ischemia and are usually followed by ST segment changes.

3. This patient should be treated with oxygen, nitrates, heparin,
   antiplatelet therapy, and statins. If he has persistent chest pain or
   elevation of cardiac biomarkers, coronary angiography may be
   indicated. Left atrial enlargement with right ventricular hypertrophy in
   this individual with a history of rheumatic heart disease may be due to
   mitral stenosis and will need further evaluation.

Case 38

38.1 Clinical Scenario

A 67-year-old male presents to your office for routine evaluation. His past medical history is significant for hypertension, hyperlipidemia, and coronary artery disease. On physical examination, he appears comfortable and in no acute distress. He is afebrile, has a heart rate of 60 beats/minute, a respiratory rate of 14/minute, and a blood pressure of 127/66 mmHg. His cardiac examination reveals a soft first heart sound and a Grade I/VI systolic murmur. You request a 12-lead ECG, a basic metabolic panel, and a lipid profile.

38.2 Questions

1. What does the ECG show?

2. What is the optimal treatment for this patient?

38.3 ECG Sample

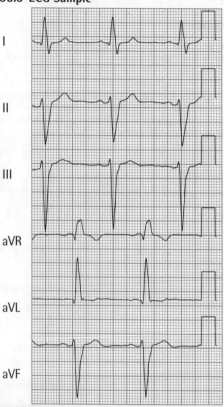

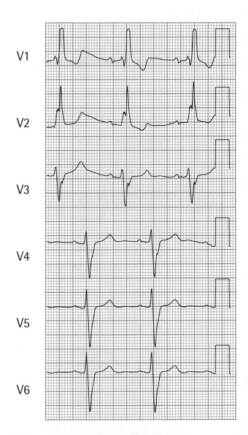

38.4 Answers

1. The 12-lead ECG shows sinus rhythm [ABIM code # 7], left anterior fascicular block [ABIM code # 45], and **complete right bundle branch block** [ABIM code # 43].

2. A bifascicular block occurs when both the right bundle branch and the left anterior fascicle are blocked. Pacing is not indicated for asymptomatic bifascicular block because the rate of progression to more advanced degrees of block is infrequent.

Case 39

39.1 Clinical Scenario

A 63-year-old male presents to your office for urgent evaluation. He states that he is having numbness and tingling sensations in the perioral area and in the fingers and toes. He also gives history of muscle cramps in the back and lower extremities and has had episodes of carpopedal spasm. His past medical history is significant for hypertension, hyperlipidemia, coronary artery disease, and recent neck surgery for a benign tumor. On physical examination, he appears irritable but in no acute distress. He is afebrile, has a heart rate of 79 beats/minute, a respiratory rate of 14/minute, and a blood pressure of 127/66 mmHg. His cardiac examination reveals a Grade I/VI systolic murmur. You request a 12-lead ECG and a complete metabolic panel.

39.2 Questions

1. What does the ECG show?

2. What is the optimal treatment for this patient?

39.3 ECG Sample

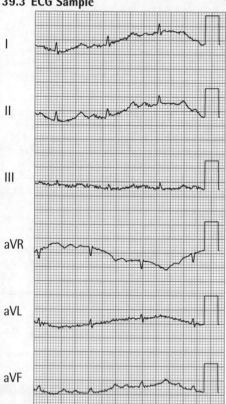

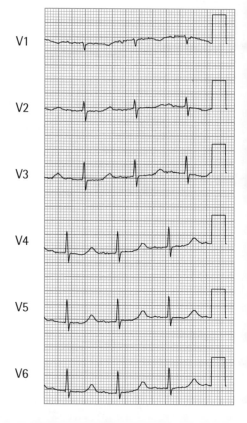

39.4 Answers

1. The 12-lead ECG shows sinus rhythm [ABIM code # 7], first-degree
   atrioventricular block [ABIM code # 29], and **hypocalcemia**
   [ABIM code # 77]. The ECG in hypocalcemia typically shows prolongation of the QT interval and repolarization changes such as
   T wave peaking or inversion.

2. Patients with hypoparathyroidism can be managed initially with the
   oral administration of calcium supplements. The hypercalcemic effects
   of thiazide diuretics may also offer some additional benefits. In patients
   with severe hypoparathyroidism, vitamin D treatment may be required.
   Parathyroid hormone deficiency impairs the conversion of vitamin D to
   calcitriol, and the most efficient treatment may be the addition of
   calcitriol or 1-alpha-hydroxyvitamin D3.

Case 40

40.1 Clinical Scenario

A 78-year-old male presents to your office with weakness, fatigue, and paresthesias. He states that he was recently started on spironolactone for heart failure. His past medical history is significant for hypertension, hyperlipidemia, and type II diabetes mellitus. On physical examination, he is in no acute distress. He is afebrile, has a heart rate of 78 beats/minute, a respiratory rate of 14/minute, and a blood pressure of 127/66 mmHg. His cardiac examination reveals a Grade II/VI systolic murmur. You request a 12-lead ECG and a complete metabolic panel.

40.2 Questions

1. What does the ECG show?

2. What is the optimal treatment for this patient?

40.3 ECG Sample

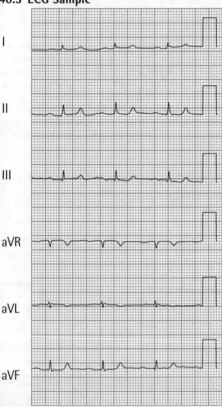

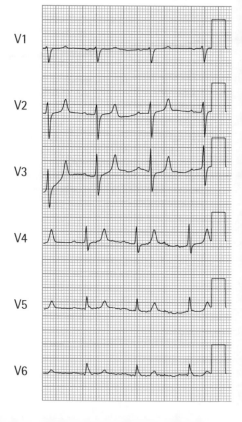

40.4 Answers

1. The 12-lead ECG shows sinus rhythm [ABIM code # 7] and peaked
   T waves consistent with **hyperkalemia** [ABIM code # 74]. Typical early
   changes of hyperkalemia include peaked T waves, shortened QT interval,
   and ST segment depression. Moderate hyperkalemia may cause bundle
   branch blocks, widening of the QRS complex, increases in the
   PR interval, and decreased amplitude of the P wave. If untreated, the
   P wave eventually disappears and the QRS morphology widens to
   resemble a sine wave. Ventricular fibrillation or asystole follows, leading
   to cardiac arrest.

2. Hyperkalemia can be treated with intravenous calcium to negate
   cardiac toxicity, glucose + insulin to increase intracellular uptake of
   potassium, and sodium bicarbonate to treat metabolic acidosis. Renal
   excretion can be increased with furosemide, and gastrointestinal
   excretion augmented by cation exchange resins such as sodium
   polystyrene sulfonate.

Case 41

41.1 Clinical Scenario

A 65-year-old male comes to your office for follow-up evaluation after a heart transplant six weeks ago. He says he is doing well and has no cardiac symptoms. His past medical history is significant for hypertension and dilated cardiomyopathy. On physical examination, he appears alert and in no acute distress. He is afebrile, has a heart rate of 79 beats/minute, a respiratory rate of 14/minute, and a blood pressure of 107/66 mmHg. His cardiac examination reveals a Grade I/VI systolic murmur. You request a 12-lead ECG and a complete metabolic panel.

41.2 Questions

1. What does the ECG show?

2. What is the optimal treatment for this patient?

41.3 ECG Sample

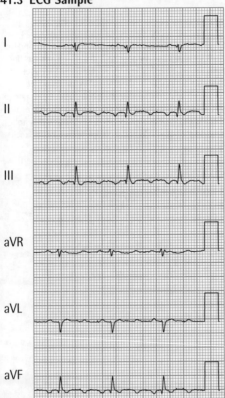

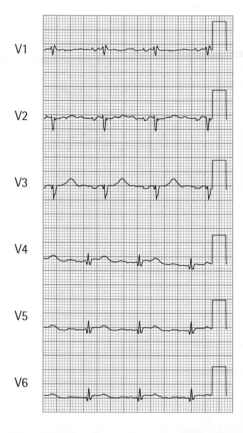

41.4 Answers

1. The 12-lead ECG shows sinus rhythm [ABIM code # 7], as well as
   atrial flutter [ABIM code # 18]. This is a unique situation seen after
   heart transplants, where two separate atrial depolarization waves may
   be seen in the surface ECG. A portion of the recipient's atria is typically
   left in situ when the donor heart is implanted, and depolarization of
   both the recipient and donor hearts may be seen on the surface ECG.

2. No treatment is necessary for this condition if the patient is
   asymptomatic and the arrhythmia is in the residual portion of the
   recipient atrium. Symptomatic arrhythmias in patients after heart
   transplantation can indirectly originate from the donor atrium via
   bidirectional recipient-donor atrial conduction and can be treated
   successfully with radiofrequency ablation.

Case 42

42.1 Clinical Scenario

A 62-year-old male comes to the emergency room with palpitations and lightheadedness that started a few minutes ago. His past medical history is significant for hypertension and prior myocardial infarction. On physical examination, he appears lethargic and diaphoretic. He is afebrile, has a heart rate of 198 beats/minute, a respiratory rate of 26/minute, and a blood pressure of 67/34 mmHg. His cardiac examination reveals a Grade I/VI systolic murmur and he has bilateral crackles on lung examination. You request a 12-lead ECG.

42.2 Questions

1. What does the ECG show?

2. What is the optimal treatment for this patient?

42.3 ECG Sample

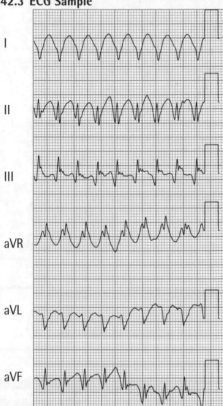

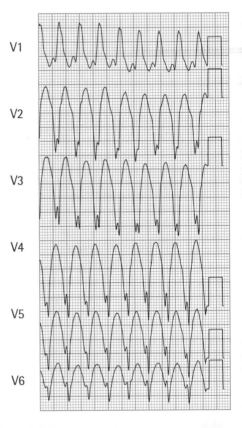

42.4 Answers

The 12-lead ECG shows sinus rhythm [ABIM code # 7], **ventricular tachycardia (VT)** [ABIM code # 25] and atrioventricular (AV) dissociation [ABIM code # 35]. VT is defined as three or more beats of ventricular origin in succession, at a rate > than 100 beats/minute. The rhythm is usually regular, but on occasion it may be modestly irregular.

ECG criteria for VT include:
- AV dissociation
- QRS axis between minus 90 degrees and plus or minus 180 degrees
- Positive QRS concordance (positive QRS V1–V6)
- QRS duration ≥ 140 milliseconds with right bundle branch block pattern and ≥ 160 milliseconds with left bundle branch block pattern
- Combination of left bundle branch block pattern and right-axis deviation
- Monophasic or biphasic QRS complex with right bundle branch block pattern and slurred or prolonged S wave in V1 with left bundle branch block morphology
- Fusion beats. Fusion beats indicate the activation of the ventricle from two foci, implying that one is of ventricular origin. When two impulses invade the ventricle simultaneously, each impulse activates that part of the ventricle, and the resulting QRS complex has a configuration that is between that of a QRS complex of the ectopic beat and the QRS complex of a sinus beat.

- Capture beats. A capture beat is the momentary activation of the ventricles by the sinus impulse during AV dissociation. During VT, the slower sinus impulse cannot be conducted antegradely to the ventricles. The sinus impulse may occasionally reach the AV node when it is no longer refractory, and is able to penetrate and capture the ventricles, resulting in a capture beat. A capture beat resembles the QRS complex of a normal sinus impulse and is preceded by a P wave. The presence of fusion beats and capture beats provides the best support for the diagnosis of VT, although they are not very commonly seen.

3. Management depends upon the hemodynamic status of the patient. VT associated with loss of consciousness or hypotension is a medical emergency requiring immediate cardioversion. This is typically accomplished with a 200–360 J monophasic shock or an equivalent biphasic energy dose. When the hemodynamic status is stable, the patient is well perfused, and no evidence for coronary ischemia or infarction is present, then a trial of intravenous medication may be considered. If left ventricular function is impaired, amiodarone or lidocaine is favored over procainamide because the potential of the latter to exacerbate heart failure. If medical therapy is unsuccessful, synchronized cardioversion is indicated.

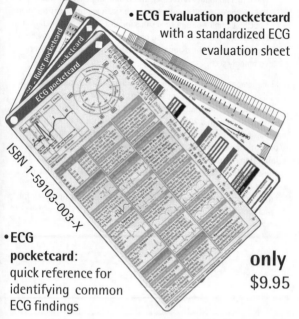

Case 43

43.1 Clinical Scenario

A 70-year-old male comes to the emergency room with palpitations and dyspnea that started two days ago. His past medical history is significant for hypertension and chronic obstructive pulmonary disease (COPD). On physical examination, he appears tachypneic and short of breath. He is afebrile, has a heart rate of 118 beats/minute, a respiratory rate of 26/minute, and a blood pressure of 167/84 mmHg. His cardiac examination reveals a Grade I/VI systolic murmur and he has bilateral crackles and rhonchi on lung examination. You request a 12-lead ECG.

43.2 Questions

1. What does the ECG show?

2. What is the optimal treatment for this patient?

43.3 ECG Sample

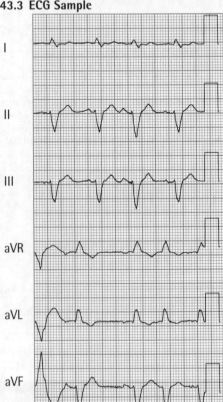

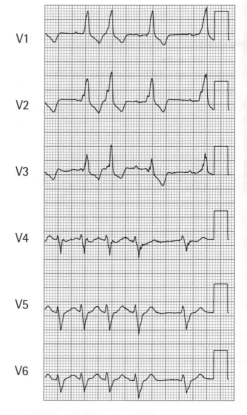

43.4 Answers

1. The 12-lead ECG shows **multifocal atrial tachycardia** (MAT) [ABIM code # 16], left anterior hemiblock [ABIM code # 45], and right bundle branch block [ABIM code # 43].

   MAT is diagnosed on an ECG when:
   - There are three or more different P wave morphologies
   - Varying P–P, PR, and R–R intervals are present
   - The atrial rate is 100–180 beats/minute
   - A narrow QRS complex is present, unless there is a conduction delay

2. MAT is most common in people admitted to the intensive care unit. MAT is usually associated with conditions that produce hypoxemia, and includes all types of respiratory failure, COPD, bacterial pneumonia, congestive heart failure, lung cancer, and pulmonary embolism.
   Any underlying condition that can precipitate MAT should be treated first. Improving oxygenation, administering intravenous magnesium, and discontinuing certain medications – such as theophylline – may be enough to terminate the MAT. Heart rate-controlling medications, such as calcium channel blockers, can be helpful.

Case 44

44.1 Clinical Scenario

A 77-year-old male comes to the emergency room with weakness and fatigue. His past medical history is significant for atrial fibrillation and he is on digoxin for rate control. On physical examination, he appears lethargic. He is afebrile, has a heart rate of 38 beats/minute, a respiratory rate of 14/minute, and a blood pressure of 79/44 mmHg. His cardiac examination reveals a Grade I/VI systolic murmur and he has bilateral crackles on lung examination. You request a 12-lead ECG.

44.2 Questions

1. What does the ECG show?

2. What is the optimal treatment for this patient?

44.3 ECG Sample

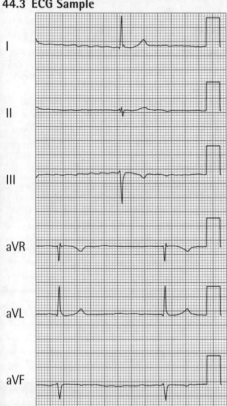

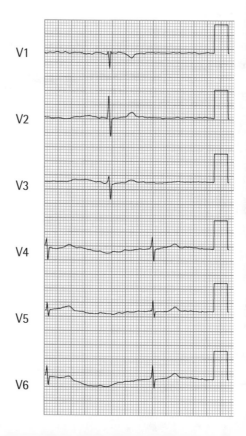

44.4 Answers

1. The 12-lead ECG shows **junctional bradycardia** [ABIM code # 21] and underlying atrial fibrillation [ABIM code # 19]. The rhythm is consistent with digitalis toxicity [ABIM code # 71].

2. The patient has symptomatic junctional bradycardia and needs a temporary transvenous pacemaker. Electrolyte alterationss, particularly hypokalemia, should be urgently corrected. Digitalis-fab antibodies (Digibind) may also be considered.

Case 45

45.1 Clinical Scenario

An 81-year-old male comes to the emergency room with weakness and fatigue for the past several days. His past medical history is significant for hypertension and prior myocardial infarction. On physical examination, he appears lethargic and disoriented. He is afebrile, has a heart rate of 34 beats/minute, a respiratory rate of 19/minute, and a blood pressure of 69/34 mmHg. His cardiac examination reveals changing intensity of the first heart sound and he has bilateral crackles on lung examination. You request a 12-lead ECG.

45.2 Questions

1. What does the ECG show?

2. What is the optimal treatment for this patient?

45.3 ECG Sample

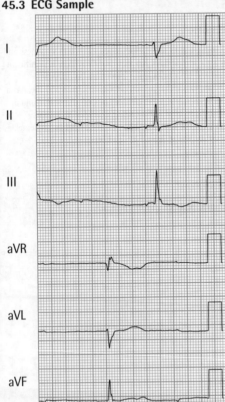

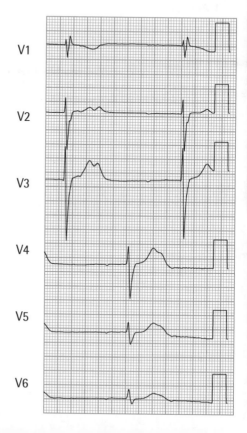

45.4 Answers

1. The 12-lead ECG shows an ectopic atrial rhythm [ABIM code # 14],
   third-degree atrioventricular (AV) block [ABIM code # 33], and a
   ventricular escape rhythm [ABIM code # 27].

2. The patient has symptomatic complete heart block and needs an urgent
   temporary transvenous pacemaker. Once he has been clinically
   stabilized, a permanent pacemaker should be considered if no
   precipitating cause is identified.

Case 46

46.1 Clinical Scenario

An 82-year-old male comes to your office with dizziness, fatigue, and generalized weakness. His past medical history is significant for hypertension and coronary artery disease. On physical examination, he appears lethargic but in no acute distress. He is afebrile, has a heart rate of 44 beats/minute, a respiratory rate of 14/minute, and a blood pressure of 108/54 mmHg. His cardiac examination reveals changing intensity of the first heart sound and he has bilateral crackles on lung examination. You request a 12-lead ECG.

46.2 Questions

1. What does the ECG show?

2. What is the optimal treatment for this patient?

46.3 ECG Sample

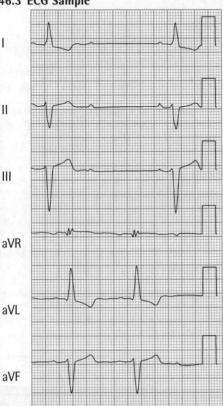

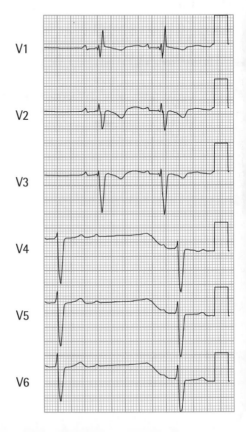

46.4 Answers

1. The 12-lead ECG shows sinus rhythm [ABIM code # 7], **second-degree atrioventricular (AV) block, Mobitz Type II** [ABIM code # 31], right bundle branch block [ABIM code # 43], and left anterior hemiblock [ABIM code # 45].

2. In Mobitz Type II block, the PR interval remains unchanged prior to the P wave that fails to conduct to the ventricles. The block is typically below the AV node, with a significant risk of progression to complete heart block. This individual with extensive conduction system disease would benefit from a pacemaker.

Case 47

47.1 Clinical Scenario

You are asked to see a 52-year-old female in the inpatient orthopedics unit for evaluation of atrial fibrillation. She recently fell and fractured her hip and is status post-hip surgery. On physical examination, she appears comfortable in no acute distress. She is afebrile, has a heart rate of 80 beats/minute, a respiratory rate of 14/minute, and a blood pressure of 122/65 mmHg. Her cardiac examination reveals normal heart sounds, without a gallop, rub, or murmur. You request a 12-lead ECG.

47.2 Questions

1. What does the ECG show?

2. What is the optimal treatment for this patient?

47.3 ECG Sample

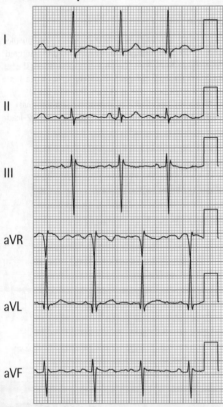

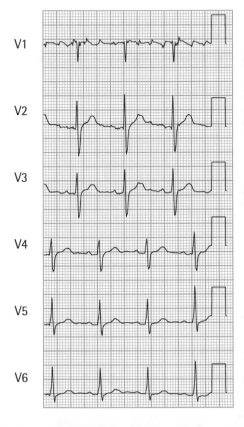

47.4 Answers

1. The 12-lead ECG shows sinus rhythm [ABIM code # 7] and **artifact** simulating atrial flutter [ABIM code # 4].

2. The patient does not have any cardiac dysrhythmia and does not need any further cardiac evaluation/treatment at this time.

Case 48

48.1 Clinical Scenario

A 62-year-old male presents to your office for cardiac evaluation. His past medical is significant for hypertension and chronic obstructive pulmonary disease. On physical examination, he appears comfortable and in no acute distress. He is afebrile, has a heart rate of 70 beats/minute, a respiratory rate of 14/minute, and a blood pressure of 129/65 mmHg. His cardiac examination reveals normal heart sounds heart sounds without a gallop, rub, or murmur. You request a 12-lead ECG and a lipid profile.

48.2 Questions

1. What does the ECG show?

2. What is the optimal treatment for this patient?

48.3 ECG Sample

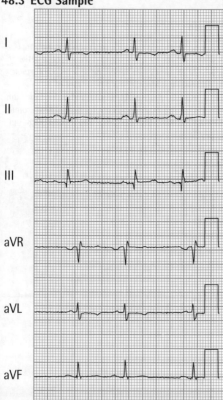

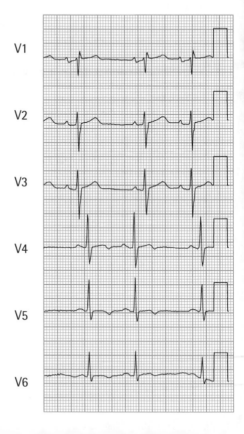

48.4 Answers

1. The 12-lead ECG shows sinus rhythm [ABIM code # 7], **3:2 SA Block, type I** [ABIM code # 12], and incomplete right bundle branch block [ABIM code # 44].

2. In type I sinoatrial (SA) block, the P-P interval shortens until one P wave is dropped (similarly to type I atrioventricular block), whereas in type II SA block, the P-P intervals are an exact multiple of the sinus cycle, and are regular before and after the dropped P wave. SA block usually occurs transiently and produces no symptoms. It may occur in healthy patients with increased vagal tone but may also be found in those with coronary disease, inferior myocardial infarction, and digitalis toxicity. This asymptomatic person does not need any treatment for his arrhythmia at this time.

Case 49

49.1 Clinical Scenario

A 73-year-old male presents to your office with palpitations. His past medical history is significant for hypertension, coronary artery disease, and heart failure. His medications include digoxin, lisinopril, furosemide, and nitrates. On physical examination, he appears comfortable and in no acute distress. He is afebrile, has a heart rate of 102 beats/minute, a respiratory rate of 18/minute, and a blood pressure of 123/65 mmHg. His cardiac examination reveals a soft, Grade I/VI systolic murmur. You request a 12-lead ECG.

49.2 Questions

1. What does the ECG show?

2. What is the optimal treatment for this patient?

49.3 ECG Sample

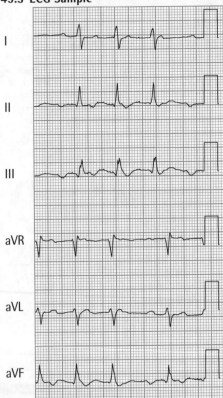

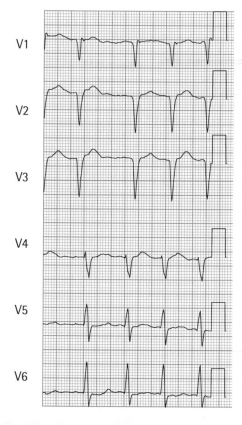

49.4 Answers

1. The 12-lead ECG shows **atrial tachycardia** [ABIM code # 15], with atrioventricular (AV) block, type I, 4:3 [ABIM code # 30], intra-ventricular conduction disturbance [ABIM code # 49], and old anteroseptal myocardial infarction [ABIM code # 54].

2. Paroxysmal atrial tachycardia, usually accompanied by 2:1 AV block, is thought to be a result of triggered automaticity. The most common cause is digitalis toxicity, which produces delayed after-depolarizations. Discontinuation of digoxin usually corrects the rhythm, and verapamil may be used for rate control, if needed.

Case 50

50.1 Clinical Scenario

You are asked to see a 56-year-old male who is admitted to the hospital for an abnormal rhythm. The patient was admitted the previous evening with an acute myocardial infarction and was treated with thrombolysis. On physical examination, he is afebrile, has a heart rate of 78 beats/minute, a respiratory rate of 18/minute, and a blood pressure of 123/65 mmHg. His cardiac examination reveals a soft, Grade I/VI systolic murmur. You request a 12-lead ECG.

50.2 Questions

1. What does the ECG show?

2. What is the optimal treatment for this patient?

50.3 ECG Sample

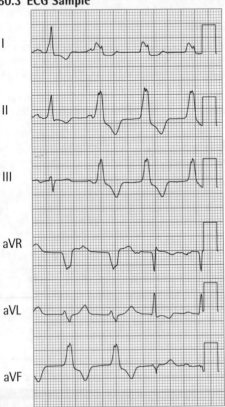

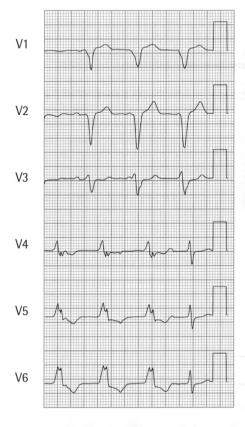

50.4 Answers

1. The 12-lead ECG shows an **accelerated idioventricular rhythm** [ABIM code # 26].

2. An accelerated idioventricular rhythm is a form of ectopic or automatic ventricular arrhythmia, characterized by a ventricular rate that is slower than traditionally defined ventricular tachycardia. Generally, the heart rate is less than 100 beats/minute and is slightly faster than the underlying sinus rhythm. Several conditions, such as myocardial ischemia, digoxin toxicity, electrolyte imbalance (e.g. hypokalemia), and hypoxemia may accentuate the phase 4 depolarization in the subordinate pacemaker tissues of the atrioventricular junction or His-Purkinje system, thus increasing the rate of impulse generation. Pharmacological or electrical suppressive therapy is rarely necessary because the rhythm is usually short lasting, the ventricular rate is generally less than 100 beats/minute, and the rate is usually well tolerated clinically.

Case 51

51.1 Clinical Scenario

A 71-year-old male presents to the emergency room with palpitations and shortness of breath. His past medical history is significant for chronic obstructive pulmonary disease (COPD, hypertension, and hyperlipidemia). On physical examination, he is afebrile, has a heart rate of 146 beats/minute, a respiratory rate of 22/minute, and a blood pressure of 113/65 mmHg. His cardiac examination reveals a soft, Grade I/VI systolic murmur and a changing first heart sound. You request a 12-lead ECG.

51.2 Questions

1. What does the ECG show?

2. What is the optimal treatment for this patient?

51.3 ECG Sample

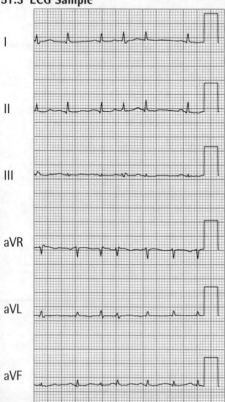

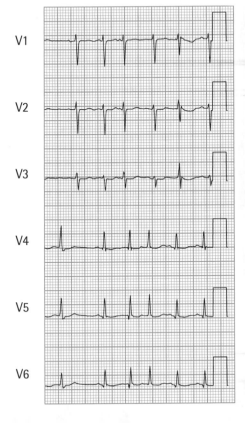

51.4 Answers

1. The 12-lead ECG shows **multifocal atrial tachycardia (MAT)** [ABIM code # 16], with functional rate-related aberrant conduction [ABIM code # 50].

2. MAT is most common in people admitted to the intensive care unit. MAT is usually associated with conditions that produce hypoxemia, and includes all types of respiratory failure, COPD, bacterial pneumonia, congestive heart failure, lung cancer, and pulmonary embolism. Any underlying condition that can precipitate MAT should be treated first. Improving oxygenation, administering intravenous magnesium, and discontinuing certain medications – such as theophylline – may be enough to terminate the MAT. Heart rate-controlling medications, such as calcium channel blockers, can be helpful.

Case 52

52.1 Clinical Scenario

A 49-year-old male presents to your office with palpitations and lightheadedness. His past medical history is significant for hypertension and hyperlipidemia. Current medications include sotalol and atorvastatin. On physical examination, he is afebrile, has a heart rate of 68 beats/minute, a respiratory rate of 16/minute, and a blood pressure of 123/69 mmHg. His cardiac examination reveals a soft, Grade I/VI systolic murmur. You request a 12-lead ECG.

52.2 Questions

1. What does the ECG show?

2. What is the optimal treatment for this patient?

52.3 ECG Sample

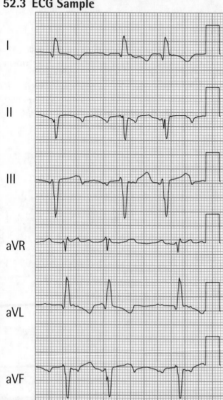

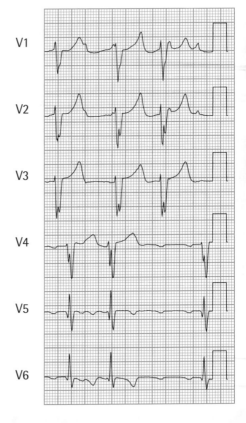

52.4 Answers

1. The 12-lead ECG shows slow **atrial flutter** [ABIM code # 18],
   intraventricular conduction disturbance [ABIM code # 49], and left
   anterior hemiblock [ABIM code # 45]. The slow flutter rate is due to
   sotalol.

2. If the patient is unstable with atrial flutter or fibrillation (e.g.
   hypotension, pulmonary edema, or angina), synchronous direct-current
   cardioversion is commonly the initial treatment of choice. Cardioversion
   often requires low energies (<50 J). If the electrical shock results in
   atrial fibrillation, a second shock at a higher energy level may then used
   to restore normal sinus rhythm. To slow the ventricular response in
   patients with tachycardia, beta-blockers or calcium channel blockers
   may be used. Adenosine produces transient atrioventricular block and
   can be used to reveal flutter waves if the diagnosis is in question. In this
   patient with a slow flutter rate and controlled ventricular rate most
   likely due to sotalol, rate control was not an issue. Most patients with
   atrial flutter can be cured with ablation. Patients with atrial flutter
   should be anticoagulated, similarly to patients with atrial fibrillation.

Case 53

53.1 Clinical Scenario

You are asked to see a 67-year-old male for an abnormal rhythm. He underwent bypass surgery three days ago and was started on sotalol on the preceding day for paroxysmal atrial fibrillation. On physical examination, he has a faint pulse with a blood pressure of 56/34 mmHg. The resident on call shows you a rhythm strip (c).

53.2 Questions

1. What does the rhythm strip show?

2. How should this patient be treated?

53.3 ECG Sample

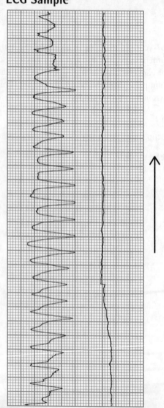

PDA software

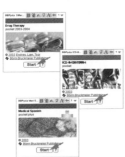

- Differential Diagnosis pocket for PDA
  (867 kb, US $ 16.95)
- Drug pocket 2005 for PDA
  (840 kb, US $ 16.95)
- Drug Therapy pocket for PDA
  (840 kb, US $ 16.95)
- ECG pocket for PDA
  (840 kb, US $ 16.95)
- Homeopathy pocket for PDA
  (2040 kb, US $ 16.95)
- ICD-9-CM 2004 pocket for PDA
  (5323 kb, US $ 24.95)
- Medical Abbreviations pocket for PDA
  (1279 kb, US $ 16.95)
- Medical Spanish pocket for PDA
  (670 kb, US $ 16.95)
- Medical Spanish Dictionary pocket for PDA
  (2343 kb, US $ 16.95)
- Medical Spanish pocket plus for PDA
  (2487 kb, US $ 24.95)

53.4 Answers

1. The rhythm strip shows **polymorphic ventricular tachycardia (VT)** [ABIM code # 25].

2. Torsade de pointes literally means "twisting of points", and is a distinctive form of polymorphic VT characterized by a gradual change in the amplitude and twisting of the QRS complexes around the isoelectric line. Torsade de pointes is associated with a prolonged QT interval, which may be congenital or acquired as a result of drug administration, as in this case. It usually terminates spontaneously but frequently recurs and may degenerate into sustained VT and ventricular fibrillation. In this hypotensive patient, immediate cardioversion is indicated. Magnesium can be used for suppressing early after-depolarizations (EADs) and terminating the arrhythmia. This is achieved by decreasing the influx of calcium, thus lowering the amplitude of the EADs. Magnesium can be given at 1–2 g IV initially in 30–60 seconds, which then can be repeated in 5–15 minutes, and appears to be effective even in patients with normal magnesium levels. Sotalol should be discontinued and temporary transvenous pacing should be considered if torsade de pointes recurs.

Case 54

54.1 Clinical Scenario

You are asked to see a 75-year-old male for pre-operative clearance prior to vascular surgery. He denies having any angina but is extremely sedentary and does minimal physical activity. On physical examination, he is afebrile, has a heart rate of 71 beats/minute, and a blood pressure of 148/79 mmHg. You request a 12-lead ECG and a complete metabolic panel.

54.2 Questions

1. What does the ECG show?

2. Does the patient need to undergo any tests prior to his elective vascular surgery?

54.3 ECG Sample

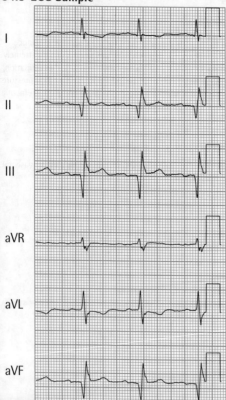

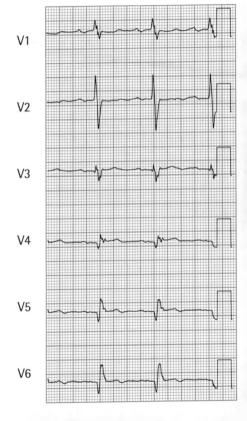

54.4 Answers

1. The 12-lead ECG shows sinus rhythm [ABIM code # 7], first-degree atrioventricular block [ABIM code # 29], deep Q waves in leads II, III, and aVF consistent with old **inferior myocardial infarction** [ABIM code # 58] and R waves in V1–V2 consistent with old **posterior myocardial infarction** [ABIM code # 60]. He also has an intraventricular conduction delay [ABIM code # 49].

2. Patients with poor functional capacity undergoing high-risk vascular surgery may benefit from non-invasive testing to further assess cardiac risk. This patient had a positive dobutamine echocardiogram, and on angiography had severe left main and three-vessel disease with a large ischemic burden. He underwent successful coronary revascularization prior to his elective vascular surgery.

Case 55

55.1 Clinical Scenario

You are asked to see a 68-year-old male for an abnormal rhythm. He had coronary artery bypass surgery three days ago. On physical examination, he is afebrile, has a heart rate of 106 beats/minute and a blood pressure of 138/79 mmHg. You request a 12-lead ECG and a complete metabolic panel.

55.2 Questions

1. What does the ECG show?

2. How should he be treated?

55.3 ECG Sample

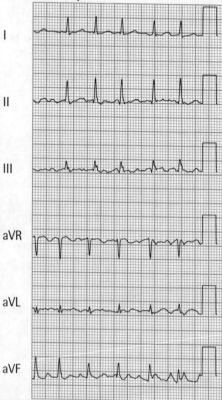

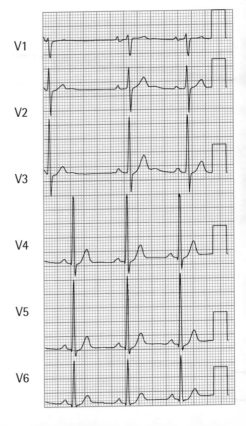

55.4 Answers

1. The 12-lead ECG shows **atrial fibrillation** [ABIM code # 19] transitioning into sinus rhythm [ABIM code # 7].

2. Beta-blockers have been clearly shown to reduce the rate of atrial fibrillation after bypass surgery and should be started in this patient. Amiodarone may be considered if beta-blocker therapy fails.

Case 56

56.1 Clinical Scenario

A 49-year-old male presents to the emergency room with crushing substernal pain. On physical examination, he is in moderate distress, is afebrile, has a heart rate of 55 beats/minute, and a blood pressure of 108/79 mmHg. You request a 12-lead ECG.

56.2 Questions

1. What does the ECG show?

2. How should he be treated?

56.3 ECG Sample

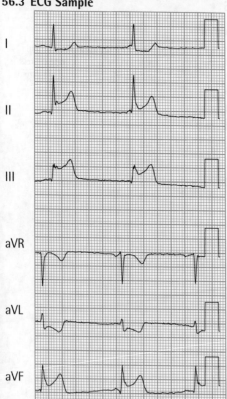

I

II

III

aVR

aVL

aVF

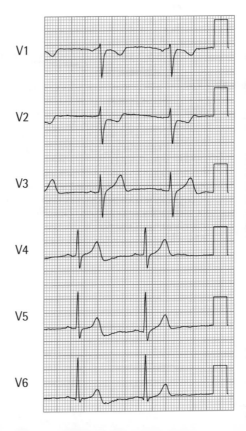

56.4 Answers

1. The 12-lead ECG shows sinus bradycardia [ABIM code # 9], acute
   inferior wall myocardial infarction [ABIM code # 57], ST segment and/
   or T wave changes suggestive of **myocardial injury** [ABIM code # 65],
   and isorhythmic atrioventricular dissociation [ABIM code # 35].

2. For patients with ST segment elevation on the 12-lead ECG, reperfusion
   therapy should be initiated as soon as possible, without waiting for
   cardiac biomarker results. This patient should preferably be sent to the
   cardiac catheterization laboratory for primary angioplasty; if such
   facilities are not available and likely transfer time is more than
   60 minutes, fibrinolytics should be administered. If immediately
   available, primary percutaneous intervention (PCI) should be performed
   in patients with ST segment elevation myocardial infarction (including
   true posterior myocardial infarction) or myocardial infarction with new
   or presumably new left bundle branch block who can undergo PCI of
   the infarct artery within 12 hours of symptom onset, if performed in a
   timely fashion (balloon inflation within 90 minutes of presentation) by
   persons skilled in the procedure

Case 57

57.1 Clinical Scenario

A 43-year-old male presents to the emergency room with palpitations and lightheadedness. On physical examination, he is dyspneac, afebrile, has a heart rate of 178 beats/minute, and a blood pressure of 78/45 mmHg. You request a 12-lead ECG. Meanwhile, his mother produces a copy of a previous ECG carried out approximately a year ago.

57.2 Questions

1. What do the ECGs show?

2. How should he be treated?

57.3 ECG Sample 1

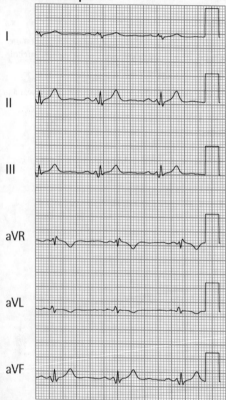

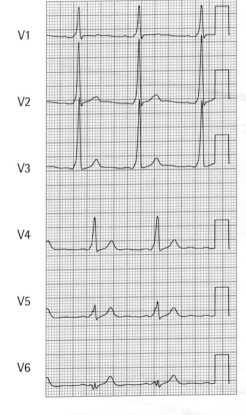

57.4 ECG Sample 2

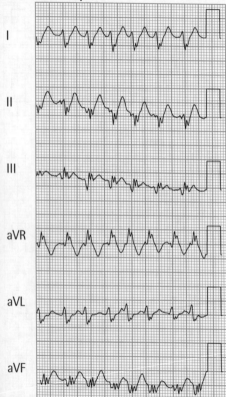

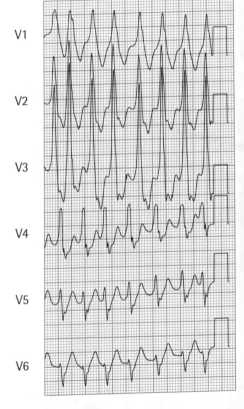

57.5 ECG Sample 3

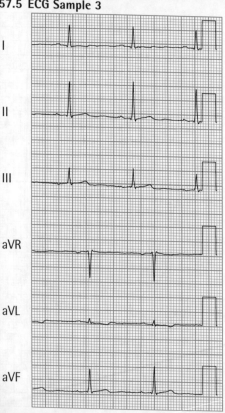

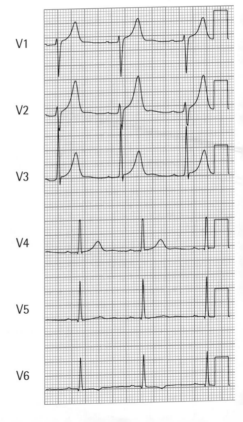

57.6 Answers

1. The baseline 12-lead ECG (a) shows a shortened PR interval, a widened
    QRS complex, and a delta wave consistent with **Wolff–Parkinson–
    White (WPW) pattern** [ABIM code # 34]. His ECG on presentation (b)
    shows atrial fibrillation with a rapid ventricular rate [ABIM code # 19].
    ECG (c) was obtained after ablation of the accessory tract, with the
    WPW pattern no longer evident.

2. WPW syndrome is the most common pre-excitation syndrome with an
    accessory atrioventricular (AV) pathway otherwise known as the Kent
    bundle. Conduction through a Kent bundle can be anterograde,
    retrograde, or both. Normal individuals are protected from exceptionally
    high heart rates during atrial fibrillation by the relatively long
    refractory period of the AV node. In patients with WPW, however, the
    accessory pathway often has a much shorter anterograde refractory
    period, allowing for much faster transmission of impulses and
    correspondingly higher heart rates and potential degeneration into
    ventricular fibrillation. If atrial fibrillation were to be treated in the
    conventional manner by drugs that prolong the refractory period of the
    AV node (e.g. calcium channel blockers, beta-blockers, digoxin), the rate
    of transmission through the accessory pathway may increase, with a
    corresponding increase in the ventricular rate. This may cause the
    arrhythmia to deteriorate into ventricular fibrillation. Procainamide
    (17 mg/kg IV infusion, not to exceed 50 mg/minute) blocks the
    accessory pathway and is the preferred agent. Prompt cardioversion of
    patients with WPW and atrial fibrillation presenting with hypotension is
    indicated. Definitive therapy is ablation of the accessory pathway.

Case 58

58.1 Clinical Scenario

A 79-year-old male presents to your office for follow-up evaluation. His past medical history is significant for heart failure and renal insufficiency. His current medications include digoxin, carvedilol, and losartan. On physical examination, he is comfortable, afebrile, has a heart rate of 73 beats/minute, and a blood pressure of 133/81 mmHg. You request a 12-lead ECG.

58.2 Questions

1. What does the ECG show?

2. How should he be treated?

58.3 ECG Sample

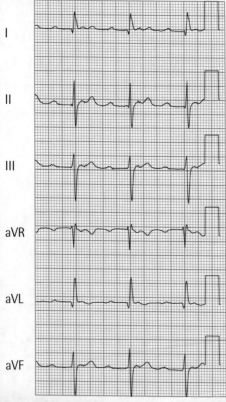

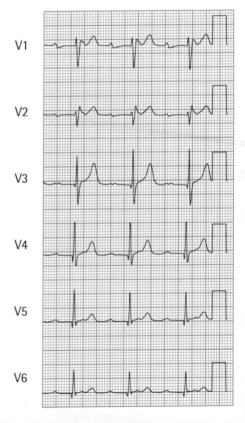

58.4 Answers

1. The 12-lead ECG shows **paroxysmal atrial tachycardia with block** [ABIM code # 15] consistent with **digoxin toxicity** [ABIM code # 71].

2. Digoxin toxicity is an important cause of atrial tachycardia, with triggered activity as the underlying mechanism. Atrial tachycardia due to digitalis intoxication often manifests with atrioventricular conduction block and/or ventricular arrhythmias. Recognizing this at an early stage is important because it may be a harbinger of more malignant ventricular arrhythmias. Treatment includes prompt discontinuation of digoxin and correction of electrolyte disturbances. The administration of antidigoxin antibodies is usually indicated in patients with high-grade conduction block, severe bradycardia, and ventricular arrhythmias. Electrical cardioversion of atrial dysrhythmias is usually not indicated because it may precipitate a ventricular tachyarrhythmia.

Case 59

59.1 Clinical Scenario

A 44-year-old female presents to your office for follow-up evaluation. Her past medical history is significant for pulmonary hypertension. She is currently taking diltiazem for pulmonary hypertension.

On physical examination, she is comfortable, afebrile, has a heart rate of 52 beats/minute, and a blood pressure of 123/69 mmHg. On cardiac examination, she has a loud second heart sound in the pulmonary area.

59.2 Questions

1. What does the ECG show?

2. What are the criteria for diagnosing this abnormality?

59.3 ECG Sample

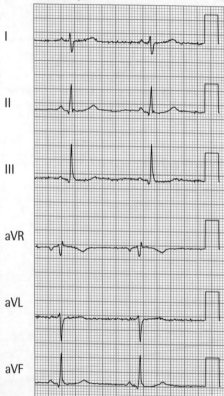

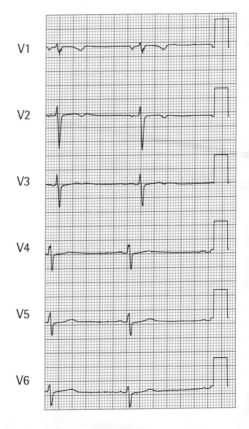

59.4 Answers

1. The 12-lead ECG shows sinus bradycardia [ABIM code # 9] and **right ventricular hypertrophy** [ABIM code # 41].

2. Right ventricular hypertrophy is commonly associated with any form of right ventricular outflow obstruction or pulmonary hypertension, which may in turn owe its origin to left-sided disease.

   ECG findings of right ventricular hypertrophy include:
   • Reversal of precordial pattern
   • Tall R in V1 and V2
   • Deep S in V5 and V6
   • Normal QRS duration
   • Late intrinsicoid deflection in V1 and V2
   • Right-axis deviation

Case 60

60.1 Clinical Scenario

You are consulted on a 74-year-old male patient in the medical intensive care unit for evaluation of his ECG changes. He was admitted with acute pancreatitis three days ago. On physical examination, he is tachypneic, febrile, has a heart rate of 104 beats/minute, and a blood pressure of 113/69 mmHg. His abdomen is markedly tender to palpation.

60.2 Questions

1. What does the ECG show?

2. What is the mechanism of this abnormality in pancreatitis?

60.3 ECG Sample

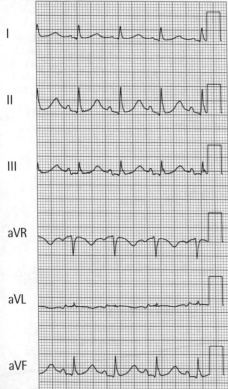

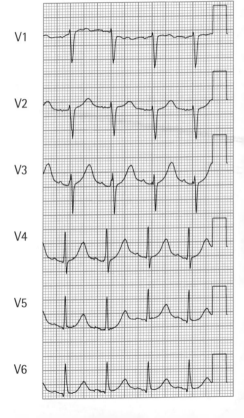

60.4 Answers

1. The 12-lead ECG shows sinus rhythm [ABIM code # 7] and changes consistent with **hypocalcemia** [ABIM code # 77]. The ECG in hypocalcemia typically shows prolongation of the QTc and ST intervals. Changes in repolarization, such as T wave peaking or inversion, can also be seen.

2. Free fatty acids chelate calcium, causing saponification in the retroperitoneum in acute pancreatitis, thus reducing calcium levels. One study suggested that relative parathyroid insufficiency may also account for the persistent hypocalcemia observed in patients with acute pancreatitis.

Index

Notes

Notes

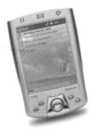

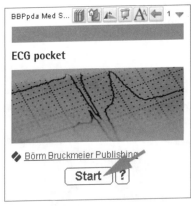

BBPpda Med S...   1 ▼

ECG pocket

◆ Börm Bruckmeier Publishing

[Start] [?]

ECG pocket for PDA
(840 kb, US $ 16.95)

- Handy reference for identifying common ECG findings
- Top-quality collection of numerous 12-lead ECGs

- Provides quick reference section and a standardized ECG evaluation sheet
- For students, residents, nurses and all other healthcare professionals

Drug pocket

For students, residents and all other healthcare professionals

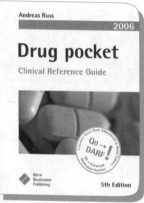

Andreas Russ

2006

Drug pocket

Clinical Reference Guide

Börm Bruckmeier Publishing

5th Edition

ISBN 1-59103-225-3   US $ 12.95

- The leading medical pocket guide, now in its fifth edition!

- Features information on more than 1,200 drugs

- Ideal for all physicians, nurses, and paramedics!

New in the 2006 edition:

- Prescription requirements and prescribing information for each individual drug

- Now includes the equation for precise calculation of dose adjustment in renal failure

- More detailed dosage information

Börm Bruckmeier Publishing
PO Box 388
Ashland, OH 44805

Börm
Bruckmeier
Publishing

Phone: 888-322-6657
Fax: 419-281-6883

Name		E-mail	
Address			
City		State	Zip

Subtotal

Sales Tax, add only for: CA 8%; OH 6.25% + Sales Tax

Shipping & Handling for US address: + S & H
UPS Standard: 10% of subtotal with a minimum of $5.00
UPS 2nd Day Air: 20% of subtotal with a minimum of $8.00

= **Total**

Credit Card: ❑ Visa ❑ Mastercard ❑ Amex ❑ Discover
Card Number

Exp. Date   Signature

For foreign orders,
quantity rebate, optional
shipping and payment
please inquire:
service@media4u.com

Books and Pocketcards also available at...   www.media4u.com

Börm Bruckmeier Products

	COPIES		PRICE/COPIES		PRICE
pockets					
Anatomy pocket		x	US $ 16.95	=	
Canadian Drug pocket 2006-2007		x	US $ 14.95	=	
Differential Diagnosis pocket		x	US $ 14.95	=	
Drug pocket 2006		x	US $ 12.95	=	
Drug pocket plus 2006-2007		x	US $ 24.95	=	
Drug Therapy pocket 2006-2007		x	US $ 16.95	=	
ECG pocket		x	US $ 16.95	=	
ECG Cases pocket		x	US $ 16.95	=	
EMS pocket		x	US $ 14.95	=	
Homeopathy pocket		x	US $ 14.95	=	
Medical Abbreviations pocket		x	US $ 16.95	=	
Medical Classifications pocket		x	US $ 16.95	=	
Medical Spanish pocket		x	US $ 16.95	=	
Medical Spanish Dictionary pocket		x	US $ 16.95	=	
Medical Spanish pocket plus		x	US $ 22.95	=	
Normal Values pocket		x	US $ 12.95	=	
Respiratory pocket		x	US $ 16.95	=	
pocketcards					
Alcohol Withdrawal pocketcard		x	US $ 3.95	=	
Antibiotics pocketcard 2006		x	US $ 3.95	=	
Antifungals pocketcard		x	US $ 3.95	=	
ECG pocketcard		x	US $ 3.95	=	
ECG Evaluation pocketcard		x	US $ 3.95	=	
ECG Ruler pocketcard		x	US $ 3.95	=	
ECG pocketcard Set (3)		x	US $ 9.95	=	
Echocardiography pocketcard Set (2)		x	US $ 6.95	=	
H&P pocketcard		x	US $ 3.95	=	
Medical Abbreviations pocketcard Set (2)		x	US $ 6.95	=	
Medical Spanish pocketcard		x	US $ 3.95	=	
Medical Spanish pocketcard Set (2)		x	US $ 6.95	=	
Neurology pocketcard Set (2)		x	US $ 6.95	=	
Normal Values pocketcard		x	US $ 3.95	=	
Periodic Table pocketcard		x	US $ 3.95	=	
Psychiatry pocketcard		x	US $ 3.95	=	
Regional Anesthesia pocketcard Set (3)		x	US $ 9.95	=	
Vision pocketcard		x	US $ 3.95	=	

Books and Pocketcards also available at...　　　　www.media4u.com